00.1

# NUTRITION AND THE
## CANCER PATIENT

# NUTRITION
# AND THE
# CANCER
# PATIENT

*Joyce Daly Margie, M.S.*

*Abby S. Bloch, M.S., R.D.*

CHILTON BOOK COMPANY

Radnor, Pennsylvania

*Designed by Adrianne Onderdonk Dudden*

*Manufactured in the United States of America*

*Library of Congress Cataloging in Publication Data*
*Margie, Joyce Daly.*
  *Nutrition and the cancer patient.*
  *Includes indexes.*
    *1. Cancer—Nutritional aspects.   2. Cancer—Diet*
*therapy—Recipes.   I. Bloch, Abby S.   II. Title.*
*[DNLM: 1. Neoplasms—Complications—Popular works.*
*2. Neoplasms—Diet therapy—Popular works. 3. Nutrition—*
*Popular works. 4. Cookery. QZ 201 M328n]*
*RC262.M323.   1983      616.99'40654      81-70351*
*ISBN 0-8019-7120-9 (pbk.)*

*1 2 3 4 5 6 7 8 9 0    2 1 0 9 8 7 6 5 4 3*

*The nutritional values used in this book were extracted from a machine-readable data base developed by Cuisine Computers Inc. (Suite 4500, 888 Seventh Avenue, New York, NY 10106) as a basis for computerized analysis of foods and recipes.*

# PREFACE

A story on the front page of the *New York Times* recently described startling scientific findings which reportedly hold out hope for "closing in fast on the secrets of cancer." This story and others like it suggest that giant strides have been made toward understanding the basic genetic factors involved in the group of diseases we call cancer. With each new discovery, it is hoped that the knowledge and understanding gained will lead to new and better ways of controlling, treating, or preventing cancer.

While this article and others like it are very careful not to promise an immediate, dramatic breakthrough, the experts do feel that cancer research is moving in the right direction and that it is moving fast.

This is good news for all those whose lives are touched by cancer—the patients themselves, their families and friends, and the numerous professionals involved in the research and treatment of cancer.

The past few decades have produced an ever-expanding body of knowledge about cancer. This increasing knowledge has led to new and better treatment methods of controlling and even curing certain types of cancer. And while neither prevention of cancer nor the perfect cure have yet been discovered, that day is coming.

In the meantime, there are many effective treatment methods currently available. Some of these treatments produce undesirable side effects, but usually these side effects are temporary and can be controlled and minimized. Among the most difficult—yet often controllable—side effects are those that affect a person's ability to obtain adequate nourishment. This can lead to additional problems since a malnourished person can lose weight, stamina, and the ability to fight disease.

This book is concerned with the nutritional and eating problems associated with cancer itself or with some of the various treatment programs used to cure or control the disease. It is our response to the mounting number of questions addressed to us, as nutritionists, both professionally and personally during the past few years. These questions have come primarily from three groups—cancer patients; family and friends of cancer patients; and medical professionals— all of whom are seeking better ways to deal with the nutritional problems caused by cancer or its treatment.

Cancer does not affect everyone in the same way; and, although not everyone with cancer develops nutritional problems, many do. Cancer patients are often urged to eat by those around them and yet they really *can't!* Appetite is often diminished; and, in some cases, there are mechanical problems that interfere with the ability to eat. Most of these problems will eventually go away, but that may not be much consolation while experiencing them.

In this book, we have attempted to give some insight into the reasons why loss of appetite, loss of taste sensations, the feeling of fullness, aversions to certain foods and aromas, and nausea before or after treatments can arise. We offer very specific, practical suggestions for dealing with these and many other nutrition-related problems. The book was written primarily for the person with cancer, but it is also intended to help serve the needs of those caring for the cancer patient: parents, spouses, relatives, friends, and medical professionals.

Background material on nutrition and the functioning of the gastrointestinal tract is provided. And there is an extensive listing of resources for additional information on various aspects of cancer in Chapter 9, as well as a list of support groups and local and national organizations dedicated to helping people with specific problems. Suggestions for increasing the calorie and protein content of recipes is given in Chapter 6. Chapters 10 to 18 contain easy to prepare recipes which have been selected to help cope with various problems that may arise.

It is not the intent of this book to answer all questions about cancer and nutrition. Rather it is intended to offer encouragement and guidance and to help solve nutritional problems which may be encountered. We hope that it will give you some insight into the reasons for nutritional problems and will provide some practical solutions to individual needs.

Ideas for recipe development were gleaned from every available source—friends, family, newspapers, magazines, food product labels, recipe booklets, and local, regional, and national cookbooks. Recipes were selected for testing and eventual inclusion in this book because they fulfilled a particular need: easy to prepare, high in calories, easy to swallow, etc. We are grateful to all the unsung cooks who unknowingly contributed to the development of this book. We are particularly indebted to the Campbell Soup Company whose ideas for making sauces from soup were so helpful.

We are grateful to the many people who helped in the development of the manuscript—Fran O'Neill, Verna Balchunas, Rosemary Arnone for the typing and retyping; Peter Engelhardt, Esq., and Health Learning Systems for the generous use of their Xerox machines for copying draft after draft; Gail Howson and the staff of the Nutrition Support Kitchen of Memorial Sloan-Kettering Cancer Center, especially Angela Sharpe and Eileen Ficco for recipe testing; Ada G. Rogers for helping gather information on pain clinics; Rachel Barcia Morse, R.D., and Mindy Hermann, R.D., and David Jacobs, M.D., for reviewing the manuscript and offering suggestions; Katherine Bergford for her excellent job of copy editing the recipes; and the patients and their families from Memorial Sloan-Kettering Cancer Center and the Summit Medical Group, Summit, New Jersey, who home-tested recipes.

We are now, and always will be, grateful to Maurice E. Shils, M.D., Sc.D., whose pursuit of excellence has served as inspiration to all who know him and whose devotion to his patients is an example to us all. And, to our families—Andrew, Paul, and Bob, who are always patient and understanding; and Darren, Renny, and especially Stan, whose continuing encouragement is appreciated more than he will ever know.

Joyce Daly Margie
Abby S. Bloch

# ACKNOWLEDGMENTS

Evelyn, John, Marylee, Edie, and Nancy, and all those with cancer whose questions and needs served as the impetus for this book.

# CONTENTS

Preface  *v*

Acknowledgments  *xiii*

## 1   Cancer and its treatment   1

What is cancer?  2

Treatment of cancer  2

Where does nutrition come in?  4

Treatment methods  5

## 2   Some background information that you might find helpful   2

Food and nutrition  10

Calories  11

Protein  13

Fats  15

Carbohydrates  15

Vitamins  16

Minerals  16

Water  17

The gastrointestinal tract  17

Digestion of food  17

Absorption of food  19

Elimination of waste products  19

## 3   Specific problems and practical solutions   20

Loss of appetite  20

Food aversions and alterations in taste and smell  22

Dry mouth  24

Sore mouth and throat  24

Feeling of fullness  25

Nausea  26

Vomiting  28

Diarrhea and cramping  29

Constipation  30

Mouth sores (stomatitis or mucositis)  31

Ostomy  31

Weight gain  32

Water retention  33

Lactose intolerance  33

Pain  34

What to do when you simply cannot eat enough  35

Tube feeding  36

Physical limitations  38

## 4   Cancer of the gastrointestinal tract   39

Cancer of the mouth, tongue and
    throat   39
Esophagus   41

Stomach   41
Small and large intestine   42
Pancreas   42

## 5   Nutrition for children with cancer   44

How cancer can affect a child's
    nutritional status   44
Nutrition program for children with
    cancer   45
Your role as a parent   47

Feeding problems and what you can
    do   48
Some nutritious snacks for
    children   51
Special reading material for children
    with cancer and their families   51

## 6   Improving the food you eat   60

Increasing calories   60
Providing extra protein   61
Adding extra nutrition to convenience
    foods   67

High-calorie and high-protein
    snacks   68
Tips for freezing food   69
Using herbs and spices   70

## 7   Some special situations you may face   72

"I just can't cope"   72
Well-meaning family and friends   73
The discomfort of those around
    you   74

No time to eat on treatment days   74
When you have to prepare food for
    your family   75
Facing an unwanted meal   76

## 8   Alternative therapies   78

Hallmarks of the charlatan   79
Mythical nutrition "cures"   81

How to protect yourself   82

## 9   Outreach: sources of help and information   84

Comprehensive cancer centers   84
Cancer information services   87
American Cancer Society   87
National and regional education and
    self-help organizations   91
Nutrition information centers   94
Pain control referral groups   94

Pain clinics, a partial listing   94
Childhood cancer programs   95
Publications from the National Cancer
    Institute   96
Other materials related to cancer and
    nutrition   98
Low-sodium information   104

## 10   Appetizers, beverages, and snacks   107

## 11   Soups, salads, sandwiches   122

## 12   Breads   137

Contents

## 13  Eggs, cheese, pasta, vegetables  145

## 14  Meats and poultry  167

## 15  Fish  189

## 16  Main dish sauces  199

## 17  Desserts  211

## 18  Dessert sauces and toppings  229

*Appendix A   Clear liquid diet   235*
*Appendix B   Moderately restricted sodium diet   236*
*Appendix C   Lactose-free diet   237*
*Appendix D   Fat-restricted diet   239*
*Appendix E   Dietary fiber content of selected foods   241*
*Appendix F   Fiber-restricted diet   242*
*Appendix G   Manufacturers of liquid formulas   244*
*Appendix H   Commercially available saliva substitutes   247*
*Appendix I   Blenderized tube feeding formulas   248*
*Appendix J   Recommended daily dietary allowances   250*

*Glossary   252*
*General index   255*
*Recipe index   262*

# NUTRITION AND THE
# CANCER PATIENT

# 1

## CANCER AND
## ITS TREATMENT

Today, because of the tremendous strides that have been made in the diagnosis, treatment, and the management of cancer, a person with cancer has good reason to be optimistic about the future. In the not so distant past, cancer was considered an acute terminal disease. But today, many cancers are considered chronic illnesses which often can be effectively treated outside the hospital. In fact, of the 3 million people in the United States who have or have had cancer, 2 million were diagnosed more than five years ago!

Today, millions of dollars are being spent in an effort to find a cure for cancer. Researchers are continually testing new and better ways of controlling cancer and when you consider that during many of our lifetimes numerous new drugs have been developed to cure or control diseases like tuberculosis, hypertension, diabetes, polio, asthma, and many infectious diseases such as pneumonia, you can understand why there is much hope that the knowledge gleaned from research will soon lead to cures for all types of cancer.

Already, these efforts have paid off. Effective treatments are now available to cure some types of leukemia and Hodgkins disease. Newly developed methods of cancer detection have led to earlier surgical intervention which also can cure some types of cancer. New chemotherapeutic drugs and advances in radiation therapy are proving very successful in arresting many other types of cancer. Sure, there are side effects of some of these new treatment methods; but in most cases they are temporary and controllable, particularly those that affect your eating patterns. That's what this book is all about—ways of maintaining your weight and sense of well being while you are undergoing anti-cancer treatments.

Today, you don't have to be a bystander—a passive recipient of treatment for a disease you wish you had never heard of. Today, you can fight back by taking an active role in your treatment program by maintaining yourself nutritionally.

## What is cancer?

Cancer is a general term used for a group of some 250 diseases distinguished by abnormal cell growth. Each type of cancer has its own name, treatment, and chances of control or cure. Despite the fact that researchers are working very hard to determine the cause of cancer, we don't have the exact answers yet. Although the causes and risk factors—which may or may not be under your control—are still being identified, cancer is still an unexplained disease.

Under normal conditions, each cell in your body develops in a very orderly fashion: when a cell wears out, it is replaced by a new cell. In cancer, a cell undergoes uncontrolled, abnormal growth—it divides two, three, four or even more times, instead of just once, and a mass (tumor) is formed. If these abnormal cells stay exactly where they are formed, the mass is said to be *localized*. If the cancer cells spread to adjoining tissues or organs or are carried by the bloodstream or lymphatic duct system to other parts of the body, the mass is described as *regional*, (confined to a specific area) or *metastasized* (spread throughout the body). Each stage is progressively more involved, so early diagnosis and prompt initiation of treatment is extremely important. Therefore, if you or someone you know suspect a problem, see a doctor right away. Early detection and proper diagnosis translate into a better chance for successful treatment.

## Treatment of cancer

Once cancer is diagnosed, it is important to learn as much as you can about cancer and its treatment. The better informed you are, the better you will be able to participate in your treatment program. Today's cancer therapy is quite specific. Very often, more than one type of therapy is used for maximum effectiveness. The type and method of treatment vary widely. Your individual program will be targeted to the stage of your disease and to the particular type of cancer you have. At the present time, the most common types of cancer treatment are *surgery, chemotherapy*, and *radiation therapy*.

No matter what your particular treatment program is, you will encounter a number of new faces. In addition to your family doctor, you will probably be seen by an *oncologist*, a physician who specializes in the treatment of cancer. And depending on the type of treatment you receive, you may have occasion to meet:

A *radiologist*, a physician with special training in interpreting X-rays.

A *radiation therapist*, a physician who has specialized training in using radiation to treat disease.

A *radiation therapy technologist*, a specially trained technician who assists the radiation therapist in giving external radiation treatments.

An *anesthesiologist*, a physician trained to administer anesthesia at the time of surgery, and in some cases consulted as a pain specialist.

A *dietitian or nutritionist*, a person with advanced specialized training in the relationship of food and nutrition to health and disease.

A *chemotherapy nurse*, a nurse who specializes in giving chemotherapy.

A *clinical nurse specialist*, a nurse who specializes in the treatment of a particular disease or health problem, such as cancer.

A *psychiatrist, psychologist, or psychiatric social worker*, mental health professionals who specialize in counselling people affected by stress or emotional problems by helping them to understand their feelings and find constructive ways of handling their problems.

An *occupational therapist*, a person with special training in the methods of treatment of convalescents, utilizing light work for diversion, physical exercise, or rehabilitation.

A *physical therapist*, a trained specialist in the treatment of disease by physical remedies such as massage and exercise.

A *pharmacist*, a medical professional who is trained in the use and preparation of drugs.

There are other hospital personnel such as medical students, residents, or fellows (graduate physicians doing advanced training) and play therapists for children—all of whom are eager to help you. If you run into a specialist with a complicated title you don't understand, ask him or her to explain his particular job to you.

Many hospital centers use a team approach to the treatment of cancer. The usual members of the team are your personal physician, an oncologist, a nurse, a dietitian, a pharmacist, and most importantly you. Other medical professionals will assist the team when they are needed. Never be shy about asking questions of the medical professionals who are helping to care for you. If you don't get an answer from one, ask another and another until you get an answer. Most will be delighted to help you and will welcome your active participation in your treatment program.

## Where does nutrition come in?

Nutrition* should be an important aspect of your overall health plan and it is particularly important when you have cancer. The old axiom "you are what you eat" certainly holds true here. If you do not make an effort to maintain yourself by eating enough of the right kinds of food, you can easily become malnourished, lose weight, feel overly fatigued, and be unable to give forth with your best efforts. And your best efforts are what you need to fight this disease. Working hard to maintain yourself nutritionally, makes you an active member of your medical team.

Research studies have shown that a person who is in good nutritional shape—that is one who is maintaining his or her ideal weight—is better equipped to withstand the rigors of the aggressive new anti-cancer therapies. Therefore, it is more important than ever that you make good nutrition part of your overall treatment.

Recent advances in the area of nutrition have proved very helpful in the management of cancer. A common and difficult problem often associated with cancer and its treatment has been weight loss. This weight loss occurs because the disease and/or its treatment can reduce appetite and food intake or interfere with your ability to consume, digest, absorb, or utilize food. Today, in most cases, thanks to the expanding body of knowledge in the field of nutrition, weight loss is not considered an unavoidable consequence of cancer. However, many people, even some medical professionals, still are unaware of the many simple and constructive steps that can be taken to ensure maintenance of body weight. In addition, exciting new feeding techniques and new and improved food products have been developed that enable almost everyone—even those

*The term nutrition refers to the process of food intake, the release of nutrients from food, and the absorption and use of nutrients by the body.

with very complicated nutritional problems—to improve their nutritional status. Unfortunately, these advances in nutrition have not been as well publicized as other advances. As a result, all too often, weight loss is still accepted as part of the disease process.

But just as with the treatment of cancer, there are no magical cures or secret solutions. Nutritional programs need to be individualized to fit each particular case. There are many things you can do on your own and this book was designed to help you and your family work with the medical professionals to produce the optimal dietary plan for you. But, you must take the primary responsibility for your own nutritional status because no one, no matter how well meaning, can "force" you to eat.

# Treatment methods

### SURGERY

Surgery was the first method used for treating cancer and it remains the primary mode of therapy. The type of cancer, its location and size, and your general overall condition are considerations in determining whether or not you should have surgery and, if so, the type of surgery you will undergo. Your nutritional status can be a critical determinant. If you are in good physical and nutritional condition, you are better able to withstand the physical demands imposed by a surgical procedure.

Surgery imposes a physiological stress by increasing your body's need for calories to supply energy and protein to rebuild damaged tissues. If you are fortunate enough to know in advance that you are going to have surgery, try to work at maintaining or regaining lost weight in order to give yourself maximum recuperative capacity. Following surgery, if you have no appetite or are unable to eat because of some mechanical problem, such as difficulty swallowing or a sore mouth, see Chapter 3 for some practical suggestions to help you. You will look better, feel better, and recover faster if you give your body the fuel it requires to meet its increased needs.

### CHEMOTHERAPY

Chemotherapy is a method of cancer treatment that employs a variety of chemical agents to destroy or impede the growth of abnormal cells. Chemotherapy may be your only treatment or it may be combined with surgery or radiation. Great advances have been made during the past few years in the use of chemotherapeutic (anti-cancer) compounds. Your physician can now select the specific drug or combination of drugs to treat your specific type of cancer cells.

Unfortunately, many people are frightened just by the word chemotherapy because they have heard stories about terrible side effects. The truth of the matter is that reactions depend on the drug or drugs being used and can vary greatly. Even people in the same treatment program can react quite differently. Some people experience few, if any, side effects; others experience a number of temporary side effects at various times during the treatment program. The majority of people who experience side effects fall somewhere in the middle, experiencing one or more temporary side effects with varying degrees of discomfort. In actuality, *only one in three people experience any side effects at all.*

The most common side effects occur in areas where there is rapid cell turnover such as in the bone marrow, hair follicles, and the lining of the gastrointestinal tract. Your doctor will monitor your therapy and check your blood frequently to detect problems caused by treatment. Many of these side effects are temporary and your doctor will adjust your therapy accordingly. Hair loss is particularly common but temporary. (Did you know hair pieces are covered by insurance?) As soon as treatment is discontinued, lost hair will be replaced by healthy new hair.

Many chemotherapeutic agents affect areas that result in either GI upset or loss of appetite. It's too easy to become malnourished if you have no appetite or have an upset stomach. Advance planning and awareness of potential problems can help you overcome possible setbacks. Some temporary nutrition-related side effects you might experience are: loss of appetite, heartburn, queasiness, vomiting, diarrhea, cramps, pain, sore mouth or throat, fatigue, weight gain, or fluid retention. Each of these is a temporary side effect and suggestions for dealing with them are contained in Chapter 3.

Queasiness, vomiting, abdominal discomfort, or diarrhea are also typical reactions to stress, and adverse reactions on the evening before or the morning of treatment are not uncommon. When you experience these types of side effects either from the chemotherapy or stress, your concern should be to meet your fluid and electrolyte*

---

*Electrolyte is a general term for the minerals necessary to create the proper environment for the body cells and to maintain the proper fluid balance in the body. Sodium and potassium are the minerals to be concerned about if you become dehydrated from excessive vomiting or diarrhea.

needs. Realistic, practical goals for such times should be: drink plenty of fluids, stick to a bland diet that will not cause gastric distress, and avoid heavy, spicy, or fatty foods that might aggravate nausea or diarrhea.

Nausea and vomiting following treatment can be minimized with a flexible, progressive eating program. Just prior to treatment stick to simple, bland, or liquid foods or refrain from eating for several hours before your treatment. On subsequent days, if you are still feeling queasy, eat soft or liquid foods that do not have strong aromas. On good days between treatments, eat foods that are loaded with calories and protein. Set priorities. Select foods that not only appeal to you but also have some nutritional value. Make every bite count so that you will get optimal nutritional value along with pleasurable eating. If vomiting is severe, ask your doctor to prescribe an anti-nausea medication.

If you feel that your gastrointestinal distress is due to stress, try to relax and refer to Chapter 4 for suggestions for dealing with various GI symptoms. If this does not help, a psychologist or psychiatric social worker may be able to suggest methods, such as relaxation or biofeedback techniques, for dealing with stress that will help you to control symptoms thereby enabling you to continue in your chemotherapy program. Ask your doctor to refer you to someone who specializes in these types of problems.

If queasiness or diarrhea lingers, refer to Chapter 3 for foods that are easy to tolerate. Don't force foods on days when you don't feel well and don't try to increase food intake until those feelings subside and you are feeling stable. However, you need to guard against losing ground by losing weight. Your nutritional state is an important factor in your ability to continue treatment and consequently in your overall future health. So, take advantage of every possible method of building yourself up when you are feeling good.

## RADIATION

Radiation used as a method of cancer treatment is a sophisticated, highly specialized methodology that employs beams of radiation, radioactive isotopes, or radioactive implants in an effort to destroy rapidly dividing cells. An impressive array of machines, each generating radiation at different energy levels, is used to treat different sizes and types of tumors while minimizing the effect on normal cells. Radiation therapy may be used alone or in combination with other treatment methods. As with chemotherapy, some people experience varying degrees of side effects; others never do.

The occurrence and degree of side effects depend on the dose per treatment, the location of the cancer, and the total amount and frequency of radiation given, as well as the individual patient's tolerance to the treatment. If radiation is directed at any part of the gastrointestinal tract, there is a potential for eating problems which in turn can lead to malnutrition.

For example, radiation to the head and neck can cause dry mouth, a sore mouth, a sore throat, or changes in taste and smell sensations, any of which can limit your food intake. Special mouth care should be instituted when you are receiving radiation to the head and mouth areas. So, as soon as you know you will be undergoing treatment in this area, visit your dentist. If your dentist is alerted beforehand, he or she can give you instructions for mouth care and can anticipate problems you may develop with your teeth, gums, or tissues in your mouth.

Another area of potential side effects is in the abdominal region. Abdominal radiation can cause nausea, vomiting, cramps, or diarrhea in some people. If symptoms are acute on the day of treatment, don't force yourself to eat; just try to maintain fluid and electrolyte intake (see footnote p. 6). Drinking broth or bouillon will help. When you feel better, increase your intake, starting with soft, bland foods and gradually progressing to your normal diet. On days when you have no side effects, try to make up for the days when you were unable to eat by selecting foods which you enjoy and which also have a high nutrient* content.

If symptoms persist or if you start to lose weight and your overall health status is deteriorating, seek professional guidance from your doctor, dietitian, or nurse. Don't wait until you have lost a great deal of weight. It is far easier to maintain your weight and sense of well being than to try to regain lost weight.


## IMMUNOTHERAPY

Another mode of treatment being used to treat some tumors is immunotherapy. This method of cancer therapy which involves stimulating the body's immune defenses attempts to utilize your

---

*A nutrient is a substance that is necessary for growth, normal body functioning, tissue repair, and maintaining life. Essential nutrients are protein, fats, carbohydrates, vitamins, trace minerals, and water.

immune system to recognize and reject abnormal, rapidly dividing cancer cells. This is a relatively new treatment method that is being carried out primarily on a research basis. A number of cancer centers are now conducting active research to determine the usefulness of this therapy and to determine the relationship between an individual's defense system and the cancerous invaders. It is hoped that this treatment method will prove to be effective in treating many types of cancer. Since it is so new, side effects and adverse reactions are not well documented. If you do experience side effects that can affect your nutritional status, check Chapter 3 under the specific symptoms you are experiencing.

# 2

## SOME BACKGROUND
## INFORMATION THAT YOU
## MIGHT FIND HELPFUL

As you read through this book, you will find two subjects that are referred to over and over again—one is food and nutrition, the other is the gastrointestinal tract with all its various parts. To help you better understand why certain recommendations concerning how you eat are being made, this chapter will briefly discuss both of these subjects.

However, no attempt is being made to provide you with an in-depth lesson in nutrition or physiology. So, if you want more information about a subject, you might want to check at your local library for books on either of these two topics.

### FOOD AND NUTRITION

As you are probably aware, nutrients are the basic fuel that the cells, tissue, and organs of your body require to reproduce, maintain, and repair themselves. Nutrition refers to that special relationship or interaction between the food you eat, the nutrients that food contains, and the effect of those nutrients on your body. Your body requires nutrients—protein, carbohydrate, fat, vitamins, minerals, trace minerals, and water—on a regular basis and in the proper amounts to help ensure that your body will function efficiently. These nutrients are absorbed through the intestinal wall and transported via your blood to individual cells throughout your body. Your cells then use the nutrients to maintain and rebuild body tissues and to perform all the necessary functions of your body. One important function is maintaining your body's natural defense system. These internal defenses help your body resist infections and are quite dependent on good nutrition.

## HOW DO YOU GET THE RIGHT NUTRIENTS?

No one food can supply all the nutrients you need each day and, unless you are thoughtfully selective, you might not be eating a good diet. To eat correctly, you need to select foods from a variety of sources so you will obtain the right balance of nutrients. To help you select a good diet and ensure that the needs of your body are being met, nutritionists (notably Dr. Frederick Stare of Harvard and his colleagues) have classified sources of nutrients into four basic food groups: meat and meat substitutes, dairy products, fruit and vegetables, and grains. Table 2-1 contains the basic four food groups and recommends the number of servings you need each day.

If you have a problem eating, you will need to pay close attention to your food intake. The need for some nutrients can be increased or modified when the body is stressed—for example, by surgery, infection, or disease. Some types of cancer may impose such a stress and you may need to adjust your intake of certain nutrients.

# Calories

In discussions concerning nutrition, the terms calories and energy are often used interchangeably. A calorie is not a nutrient as such, it is a measure of energy. The nutrients that supply the energy or calories needed to sustain life are protein, fat, and carbohydrate. Each of these nutrients contributes a specific number of calories based on gram weight to your total intake.*

Individual calorie requirements vary, depending on such factors as age, body size, metabolic rate, and the level of physical activity. Ideally, calorie intake balances calorie expenditure and your body weight remains constant. However, that is not always the case and many of us have learned first hand that the intake of excess calories

---

*Fat provides nine calories per gram, protein and carbohydrate each provide four calories per gram. One ounce is equal to approximately 28 grams.

## TABLE 2-1 BASIC FOUR FOOD GROUPS

| | Foods in this group | Major nutrients supplied | Recommended servings | Serving size |
|---|---|---|---|---|
| Meat and meat substitutes | Beef, pork, veal, lamb, fish, poultry, eggs, organ meats, cheeses, dry beans, lentils, peas, nuts. | Protein, fat, niacin, iron, thiamine, vitamin $B_{12}$, vitamin E, phosphorus, copper | Adults, children, teenagers, 2; pregnant and nursing women, 3 | 2 ounces cooked meat, fish, poultry; 2 eggs; 1 cup cooked dry beans, peas, lentils; $\frac{1}{2}$ cup nuts; 4 tablespoons peanut butter; 2 ounces hard cheese; $\frac{1}{2}$ cup cottage cheese; 2 cups milk may be substituted for one serving of meat. |
| Dairy | Milk, yogurt, natural and unprocessed cheeses, ice cream, ice milk, other food products made with milk | Protein, fat, calcium, riboflavin, vitamins A and D, magnesium, zinc | Children, 3; teenagers, 4; adults, 2; pregnant and nursing women, 4. | 1 cup milk or yogurt; 1 ounce cheese; $\frac{1}{2}$ cup cottage cheese; $\frac{1}{2}$ cup ice cream; 1 cup milk-based product (pudding, soup, or beverage). |
| Fruits and vegetables | All fruits and vegetables (fresh, frozen, dried, canned) and juices. | Carbohydrates, water, vitamins A and C, iron, magnesium. | Everyone, 4 (including 1 citrus fruit daily and 1 deep green or yellow vegetable every other day). | 1 cup cut-up raw fruit or vegetable; 1 medium apple, banana, orange, tomato, potato; $\frac{1}{2}$ melon or grapefruit; $\frac{1}{2}$ cup cooked vegetable or fruit, $\frac{1}{2}$ cup fruit or vegetable juice. |
| Grains | Wholegrain or enriched white flour, pasta, rice, cereal products. | Carbohydrate, fat, protein, thiamine, niacin, vitamin E, calcium, iron, phosphorus, magnesium, zinc, copper. | Everyone, 4. | 1 slice bread; 1 ounce dry cereal; 1 roll or muffin; 1 pancake or waffle; $\frac{1}{2}$ cup rice, pasta, cooked cereal. |

CALORIC EXTRAS: Except for fats, the following foods have little nutritional value, so no specific amount is recommended. They should be added to your diet in the amounts required to maintain the appropriate caloric allowance for you: Butter, margarine, shortening, oils, dressings, condiments, sugars, candies, syrups, jams, unenriched refined grain products, sweetened desserts and pastries, soft drinks, and presweetened fruit drinks.

*Nutrition and the Cancer Patient*

results in weight gain and conversely that the intake of insufficient calories will lead to weight loss.

Your body has a paramount requirement for calories to meet its energy demands for basic body functions. Before any other body need can be met, the need for calories must be satisfied, even if it means your body must use its own tissues to supply the necessary calories. When you eat less or cannot utilize food efficiently, your energy needs cannot be met. If this continues for an extended period of time, you will begin to show signs of starvation. Your body will begin to use muscle protein and fat stores as sources of energy. Tissues will become increasingly smaller and even organs such as the liver, kidney, and heart will eventually be affected. A weakened, malnourished body will be unable to carry on everyday functions, much less fight disease.

To estimate your daily calorie needs, adults (see Chapter 5 for children) can use the following rule of thumb: multiply your desired weight in pounds by 14 to 16 depending on your activity level. If you are:

sedentary, multiply by 14
moderately active, multiply by 15
active, multiply by 16

If you are underweight, you should add at least 500 calories a day until you have gained lost weight.

If you are very active, add extra calories.

If you don't know what your weight should be, see Table 2-2.

The best food sources of calories are fats followed by carbohydrates. Proteins should be reserved for tissue building and not used to meet basic energy needs unless absolutely necessary.

## Protein

The protein in your food provides amino acids which are used by your body to build and repair tissues, to create antibodies to fight infection, and to assist in numerous body functions. If you don't consume enough calories from fat and carbohydrate sources to meet your energy needs, your body will be forced to use protein to meet its energy needs and the building and repair functions of protein will be shortchanged.

In most cases, protein requirements are easily met because they are not excessively high. If you are consuming enough calories to

## TABLE 2-2  HEIGHT AND WEIGHT STANDARDS

Following are 1983 weight tables by height and size of frame, for people aged 25 to 59, in shoes and wearing five pounds of indoor clothing for men, three pounds for women.

### MEN

| Height | Small | Medium | Large |
|--------|-------|--------|-------|
| 5'2" | 128–134 | 131–141 | 138–150 |
| 5'3" | 130–136 | 133–143 | 140–153 |
| 5'4" | 132–138 | 135–145 | 142–156 |
| 5'5" | 134–140 | 137–148 | 144–160 |
| 5'6" | 136–142 | 139–151 | 146–164 |
| 5'7" | 138–145 | 142–154 | 149–168 |
| 5'8" | 140–148 | 145–157 | 152–172 |
| 5'9" | 142–151 | 148–160 | 155–176 |
| 5'10" | 144–154 | 151–163 | 158–180 |
| 5'11" | 146–157 | 154–166 | 161–184 |
| 6'0" | 149–160 | 157–170 | 164–188 |
| 6'1" | 152–164 | 160–174 | 168–192 |
| 6'2" | 155–168 | 164–178 | 172–197 |
| 6'3" | 158–172 | 167–182 | 176–202 |
| 6'4" | 162–176 | 171–187 | 181–207 |

### WOMEN

| Height | Small | Medium | Large |
|--------|-------|--------|-------|
| 4'10" | 102–111 | 109–121 | 118–131 |
| 4'11" | 103–113 | 111–123 | 120–134 |
| 5'0" | 104–115 | 113–126 | 122–137 |
| 5'1" | 106–118 | 115–129 | 125–140 |
| 5'2" | 108–121 | 118–132 | 128–143 |
| 5'3" | 111–124 | 121–135 | 131–147 |
| 5'4" | 114–127 | 124–138 | 134–151 |
| 5'5" | 117–130 | 127–141 | 137–155 |
| 5'6" | 120–133 | 130–144 | 140–159 |
| 5'7" | 123–136 | 133–147 | 143–163 |
| 5'8" | 126–139 | 136–150 | 146–167 |
| 5'9" | 129–142 | 139–153 | 149–170 |
| 5'10" | 132–145 | 142–156 | 152–173 |
| 5'11" | 135–148 | 145–159 | 155–176 |
| 6'0" | 138–151 | 148–162 | 158–179 |

*Source:* Metropolitan Life Insurance Company, 1983.

meet your energy needs, one-half gram protein per pound of body weight is more than sufficient for an average adult. However, your protein requirements may be higher if treatment or disease has caused extensive tissue damage or muscle wasting.

Meat, fish, poultry, eggs, milk, cheese, nuts, dried beans, and peas are all good sources of protein. It is fairly easy to add protein to your diet without forcing yourself to eat large amounts of food. For example, you can use milk instead of water in cooking hot cereal, add melted cheese to rice, pasta, or potatoes, and incorporate eggs into recipes whenever possible. Chapter 6 will give you some suggestions for increasing the protein content of a recipe.

## Fats

Fat supplies the calories necessary for warmth and physical work. In addition, the fat in your food provides "essential fatty acids" which are needed for growth, hormone production, cell membrane structure, and transportation of vitamins (A, D, E, K) which are not soluble in water. Your body stores excess calories as fat. Stored fat acts not only as a reserve energy source but also insulates your body against rapid shifts in temperature and pads your vital organs and nerves to protect them against trauma.

In general, the requirements of fat (other than for calorie needs) are very low. Yet fat accounts for approximately 30 to 40 percent of the calories in most Americans' diets. Fat is a more concentrated source of calories than either protein or carbohydrate. Therefore, if you need to increase your calorie intake, fat is a good, easy choice. However, some people find it difficult to consume fat in quantity because fat seems to decrease their appetite or to be hard to digest. The main food sources of fat are butter, margarine, vegetable oil, shortening, salad dressing, fatty meats, whole milk products, cream, and nuts. If you need to increase the calories in your diet, check Chapter 6 for some ideas for adding various fats to your food.

## Carbohydrates

Your body uses carbohydrates to supply energy for heat and to do the mechanical work of your body. Carbohydrate foods, such as fruits, vegetables, and whole grain products also contribute valuable vitamins, minerals, and fiber to your diet.

Carbohydrates are relatively inexpensive and readily available sources of calories. Carbohydrate foods should account for about 50% to 60% of your total calorie intake each day. Good sources of carbohydrate are fruits, vegetables, starches, flours, grains, pasta, and in sugars like honey, molasses, syrups, and table sugar. These latter sources of concentrated carbohydrate can add significant calories to your overall intake without adding much extra bulk to your diet, but do not contribute any other nutrients.

## Vitamins

Vitamins regulate or take part in many of the metabolic processes and biochemical reactions that take place in your body. The best way to get the vitamins you need is to eat a varied diet containing lots of fruits and vegetables. However, if you don't have much of an appetite, try combining fruits and vegetables with other foods so you will be able to meet your calorie requirements. For example, you can add vegetables to egg dishes or casseroles or prepare them with extra butter or a cream sauce. You can top fruits with whipped cream or serve with ice cream and a high calorie topping.

Vitamin requirements are outlined in a chart in Appendix J. If you feel that you are unable to eat enough food to meet the recommended daily allowances of vitamins, ask your doctor whether he or she recommends a multivitamin supplement. In many cases, vitamin requirements are not increased by cancer or its treatment; and despite extravagant claims, there is not enough scientific evidence to date that megadoses of vitamins have therapeutic effects on cancer. In fact, in some instances, large doses of vitamins may interfere with your treatment. So, check with the physician in charge of your treatment before you start taking any vitamin supplement. In fact, you should make it a rule to check with your physician before starting any new medication, whether it is prescribed by another physician or purchased over the counter since any one could possibly effect your treatment in some way.

## Minerals

Minerals are essential nutrients in your diet because they are needed to activate, regulate, and control many of the metabolic functions that take place in your body. And, just as with vitamins, the required amounts of most minerals can be supplied by eating a variety of foods from the basic four food groups. So unless your physician specifies that you need supplements, you are probably getting enough if you eat a balanced diet. However, if you are not eating very much, you may be a candidate for iron or other mineral supplements. But be sure to check with your doctor before taking any supplements.

## Water

Water makes up one-half to two-thirds of your total body weight. Water is necessary to regulate body temperature, to carry nutrients to their sites of action, to carry away metabolized waste products, and to bathe the cells. Unless you have been instructed to reduce your fluid intake, try to drink six to eight glasses a day even when you are not feeling well. If you have a poor appetite, high calorie liquids should be substituted for water.

Be sure to follow your doctor or pharmacist's instructions concerning fluid intake since some chemotherapeutic agents increase your need for water.

## THE GASTROINTESTINAL TRACT

The gastrointestinal (GI) tract (see Fig 2-1) consists of all those parts of your body that are involved in the digestion and absorption of food. The work of the GI tract starts when you put food in your mouth and ends with the elimination of waste products. Unfortunately, in some cases, cancer and its treatment can be accompanied by problems which affect the GI tract. And any problems that affect the GI tract potentially can have an adverse effect on your nutritional status. Therefore, it is helpful for you to know a little about the GI tract. Then if you do develop a problem, you will have a better understanding of what is happening and be better prepared to deal with it.

## Digestion of food

The process of digestion starts in your mouth where the food is reduced into smaller pieces by your teeth, and saliva begins to dissolve and lubricate it. The starch-digesting enzyme in saliva also begins the breakdown of starches into simpler sugars.

When food leaves your mouth, it is swallowed through the pharynx, or throat, and is pushed along through your esophagus by

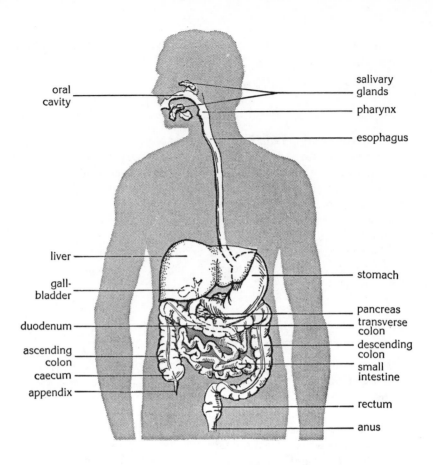

oral cavity

salivary glands

pharynx

esophagus

liver

stomach

gall-bladder

pancreas

duodenum

transverse colon

ascending colon

descending colon

caecum

small intestine

appendix

rectum

anus

coordinated, wave-like contractions called peristaltic movements. Just before the food enters your stomach, it passes through a special valve designed to keep the stomach contents from flowing back into the esophagus.

Once in the stomach, the food is homogenized and mixed with enzyme containing gastric juices. These juices then begin the break down of protein into its simplest form—amino acids. Some fat digestion also takes place in the stomach. Carbohydrates, which require little digestion, pass relatively quickly through the stomach.

The pancreas, liver, bile ducts, and gall bladder all play important roles in the digestive process. The pancreas secretes water, bicarbonate, and digestive enzymes into your intestine and provide the insulin and glucogen necessary for carbohydrate regulation and metabolism. The liver turns the protein you eat into usable body protein, converts nutrients into energy, stores carbohydrates and some fats and protein, and produces bile salts needed by your body for digestion and absorption of fat. The bile ducts carry the bile manufactured in the liver to the gall bladder, where it is stored until needed for the digestion of fat in your small intestine.

## Absorption of food

Upon leaving the stomach, food enters the small intestine where any remaining protein, starch, and fat are digested by bile, and the pancreatic and bowel enzymes. After your food is digested and hydrolyzed into its simplest nutrient forms—peptides, amino acids, fatty acids, simple sugars, vitamins, minerals—the nutrients are absorbed into your bloodstream and transported throughout your body where they are used to nourish all cells of your body. Ninety to ninety-five percent of nutrient absorption takes place in the jejunum, part of the small intestine.

The lining of your small intestine is not smooth. It is made up of millions of finger-like folds called villi, which in turn have millions of hair-like projections called microvilli. The purpose of the villi and microvilli is to increase the surface of the intestinal lining so that nutrients can be effectively and rapidly absorbed. The lining of your small intestine is one of the areas in your body where there is a very rapid turnover of cells. In other words, the cells on the surface of your small intestine are replaced more often than in many other parts of your body. For this reason, these cells are very sensitive to cancer therapy.

## Elimination of waste products

Fiber and the unabsorbed products of digestion continue into your large intestine, or colon. The primary function of the colon is to reabsorb most of the water that was secreted into the GI tract to assist in the digestive process. If this water is not reabsorbed, you could develop diarrhea and become dehydrated. The waste products of the digestive process are held in your rectum which is located at the end of your colon until they are eliminated, thus ending the digestive and absorptive processes.

# 3

## SPECIFIC PROBLEMS AND
## PRACTICAL SOLUTIONS

The nutritional problems associated with cancer and its treatment are many and varied, but they are not cause for despair. In most cases, they are manageable. Furthermore, you may not encounter any of the complications described in this chapter. Contrary to popular belief, only one person in three experiences side effects from therapy, and most of these effects are temporary, particularly those caused by treatment.

The best approach to managing side effects is a direct one. Bring out your problem-solving skills. Observe your progress carefully, and learn to recognize problems when they first surface. Don't try to ignore them and carry on. Face them and cope. Whatever the cause, you will minimize the effects and make better headway against the disease by keeping yourself well-nourished.

## Loss of appetite

Anorexia, or loss of appetite, is frequently associated with chronic disease. In addition to treatment, there are two underlying causes for anorexia in cancer.

The first is somewhat mysterious: Many people experience a loss of appetite long before there is any medically detectable symptom of cancer. At the present time, some believe this phenomenon may be the body's reaction to abnormal cell growth. Whatever the reason, this decrease in appetite causes many to be underweight and rundown when they first present themselves to a doctor for diagnosis. The weight should be regained as soon as possible.

Anxiety and depression are common causes of decreased appetite and weight loss under any circumstances. It is normal to experience some degree of anxiety or fear for a day or two before a visit to a doctor or dentist. These feelings are heightened at the first hint of a serious health situation or at the initial diagnosis of cancer. When the anxiety is prolonged—for example, during the period of an initial diagnostic work-up—weight loss is not uncommon. This is probably the lowest emotional point in the whole disease process— adjusting mentally to the harsh reality; fighting denial, fear, defeatism, and perhaps the unjustified guilt that often comes with serious illness; and reevaluating life priorities. It is a wrenching, intense experience that can be surmounted only by acceptance of your condition. The single best thing you can do—the life-affirming gesture—is to nurture yourself by nourishing yourself. Reverse the weight loss, and participate wholeheartedly in your treatment therapies.

## Suggestions

Your goal is to eat enough calories, protein, and other essential nutrients to meet your basic needs and maintain your weight. Do whatever is most convenient and works best for you.

*If you are not hungry at dinner time,* make breakfast, midmorning snacks, and lunch your main meals and don't worry about dinner.

*If you don't feel like eating in the morning,* have a light snack, and eat later in the day when you feel better.

*Don't feel locked in to the conventional meal pattern.* It is not necessary to eat three large meals; several small meals spread throughout the day can achieve the same nutritional goals.

*Make the food you eat count.* There is nothing to be gained by sitting down to a large plate of food you don't want to look at, much less eat. Try a "Meal-in-a-Glass" or high-calorie snacks (see Chapter 10). Taking just a few bites or a sip of the right food every hour or so can make a significant contribution to your total calorie and/or protein intake.

*Check the recipe section for dishes that appeal to you.* Calorie and protein contents are given, so you can select recipes that maximize calorie intake in small portions.

*Use the suggestions in Chapter 6 to augment protein and calorie intake.*

*If your appetite loss is caused by queasiness or nausea,* eat small portions. Try to eat dry foods like crackers or bread to settle your stomach in the morning. Later in the day, when you feel better, concentrate on foods that are not spicy or high in fat. (See the section on Nausea in this Chapter.)

*If you cannot keep your mind off your problems,* eat with others to divert yourself. You may well find you are able to relax and enjoy your meals more if you socialize with family and friends.

*A glass of wine, beer, or a cocktail* before lunch or dinner can help to increase your appetite if there is no contraindication (check with your physician). Alcohol is also a good source of extra calories.

*Do not stop eating because you have lost your appetite.* Make a concentrated effort to eat even when you are not hungry. Overcoming anorexia is a matter of trial and error. Develop a program that will work for you, and revise it if necessary as you go along. Some people simply work out an eating schedule and stick to it no matter what, because, quite rightly, they look at eating as an important part of their treatment program and as an investment in their future.

*If you are in the hospital,* have your family or friends bring in your favorite foods, or ask your doctor if it is possible to go out for dinner occasionally.

*Think of eating as an essential part of your treatment program.*

## Food aversions and alterations in taste and smell

Researchers have suggested that alterations in taste and odor sensation may be the result of metabolic changes, but anxiety also appears to cause this reaction in some. At any rate, many people who have cancer report that food "just doesn't seem to taste right" or that certain foods no longer agree with them or no longer appeal to them. Some report an aversion to meat, coffee, or chocolate. Others have an elevated taste threshold for bitterness; or report metallic, cottony, or strange tastes; or encounter decreased taste threshold for sweetness.

In most cases, these alterations in taste are real and probably represent a response to changes the body is undergoing as a result of the disease or the treatment.

Some types of chemotherapy and radiation cause these changes and radiation to the head and neck can also result in "mouth blindness", a loss of taste.

If some foods lose their appeal for you, concentrate on selecting the ones you now enjoy. There are so many choices available that you should still be able to meet your nutritional needs. Don't force yourself to eat anything that doesn't seem appetizing.

## Suggestions

*As a first step, check with your dentist* to rule out any dental problems which might be causing a bad taste in your mouth or otherwise altering your taste. Your dentist will also be happy to recommend special mouth care and mouthwashes that may help.

*Next ask your doctor about your medications.* If you are taking a drug that is causing changes in taste sensation, it may be possible to change the medication or the dosage.

*If you develop a strong dislike for a food* or find that a particular food, like beef, grapefruit, or coffee tastes strange to you, simply eliminate the offending item and substitute one of similar nutrient value.

*Use wines, salad dressings, and strong seasonings* in cooking. Adding strongly flavored juices or relishes can also improve the taste.

*Try cooking and serving with plastic* rather than metal utensils to reduce the bitter taste of food.

*If red meat begins to taste bitter,* and you lose your appetite for beef, lamb, or pork, soak or cook it in soy sauce, fruit juice, or wine, or marinate it before cooking.

*If sauces and marinades don't do the trick,* substitute other foods high in protein—chicken, turkey, eggs, fish, high-protein puddings, ham, custards, peanut butter, ice cream, milkshakes, yogurt, cheese, peas, beans, nuts, or macaroni and cheese, a fine old standard which seems to maintain its appeal for many who are chronically ill.

*If your taste perception is dulled,* try to intensify the aroma of food, and eat food with distinctive textures to get more satisfaction from eating.

*To overcome a metallic taste,* eat lemons or other tart fruits or fruit-flavored sour balls.

*Experiment with changing the temperature of food.* Frequently, foods that taste "skewed" warm or at room temperature will taste better to you chilled or frozen.

*Be adventuresome.* Change not only the temperature of food but the taste. If you do not have soreness or discomfort in your mouth, very spicy, salty, or tart, unsweetened food may be more savory than traditionally seasoned food. Try changing a food that would normally be sweet to a tart or tangy taste. Don't be concerned if others turn up their noses. You are the one you have to please.

# Dry mouth

Another taste-related problem some encounter is "dry mouth." It may be caused by a drug or medication or by treatment. Some treatments, such as radiation to the oral cavity, can affect the ability to produce saliva.

## Suggestions

*Eat soft foods* that are easy to swallow, and add gravies, sauces, salad dressing, broth, sour cream, or mayonnaise to make them moist.

*Use artificial saliva.* There is a variety of topically active oral rinses and lozenges to moisten and lubricate the mouth. However, several new sprays now commercially available are significantly more long-lasting and effective than the rinses and lozenges. Ask your dentist or doctor about them. (See Appendix H.)

*Chew sugar-free gum or suck on ice chips* to help keep your mouth moist.

*See the Recipe section for sauces* that can be used on meats, vegetables, or desserts to help moisten your mouth as you eat. Most soups and casserole dishes are easy to swallow.

*Drink liquids with your meals.* Be sure they are high-calorie liquids if you need to gain weight.

*Cold foods* are often better tolerated than warm or hot ones.

*Dunk dry foods*, like bread, in a soup or beverage to moisten them.

*Concentrate on highly nutritious liquids* like blender meals (see page 117) and liquid complete nutritional supplements (see Appendix G).

# Sore mouth and throat

Some types of treatment can cause a sore mouth or throat, not unlike the sensation encountered with a bad cold or a strep throat which makes swallowing difficult. This is uncomfortable, but it is not insurmountable.

## Suggestions

*Try to eat a variety of soft, easy-to-swallow foods,* such as soups, eggs, flaked fish, pastas, quiches, souffles, cheese dishes, dairy products, and liquid meals, all of which can provide good nutrition with a minimum of discomfort in the passage through the mouth and throat.

*Try stewing meat* instead of broiling or frying it.

*Avoid* highly seasoned, spicy, tart, or acidic foods which are often irritating, as are cigarette smoking and alcoholic beverages.

*Cut food into very small pieces.*

*If it is difficult to chew bite-size pieces,* try mashing, blending, straining, or pureeing food, or try baby foods.

*Make a deliberate effort to keep your calorie intake up* by concentrating on high-calorie, high-protein beverages and soups (see recipe section).

*Moderate the temperature of food.* Eat things that are cold or at room temperature.

*If you have trouble swallowing,* try using a straw for beverages and a cup or glass instead of a spoon for liquids like soup.

*If swallowing is extremely difficult,* ask your doctor for a referral to an occupational therapist who can help you locate specialty equipment such as special utensils, or to a speech therapist who can teach you new swallowing techniques.

*If brushing your teeth is painful,* you can clean them with a cotton swab dipped in a half-and-half solution of warm water and 3% hydrogen peroxide.

*Ask your physician about anesthetic lozenges and sprays* that can numb the mouth and throat long enough for you to eat your meal.

*After meals reduce irritation from abrasive or acidic food* (citrus fruits or tomatoes) by rinsing your mouth with a baking soda or bicarbonate of soda solution (one teaspoon soda to one cup warm water).

## Feeling of fullness

Early satiety—feeling full after having eaten a small amount of food—has a number of different causes. Anyone can experience physical reactions such as an upset stomach, loss of appetite, and early satiety when under stress or preoccupied with problems. In cancer therapy, medication or treatment can sometimes cause you to feel full—as if you "simply don't have any room." Constipation can also induce these symptoms because the body is not ridding itself of previously eaten foods. The tips that follow will help you coax yourself to eat.

### Suggestions

*Eat small amounts of food* six to eight times a day.

*Make sure these mini-meals are high in nutrient density,* so the sum total of your daily intake meets your nutritional goals. For example, if you feel you can only eat two or three mouthfuls of solid food, don't rely on Jell-O, salad, or a piece of fruit. Select concentrated sources of calories and proteins. See the section on increasing the nutrient density of foods (in Chapter 6) and the recipe section for suggestions.

*Drink fluids after solid food* has been consumed. Any liquids— water, fruit juices, or clear broth—fill you up and decrease your capacity for solid food. If you must drink some fluid to make your meal more palatable and to help you swallow, drink nutritionally significant ones like milk, cream or hearty soups, or eggnog.

*Exercise between meals* if you are able. Taking a short walk can go a long way toward helping you digest your food.

*Approach meals in a relaxed manner.* Unwind before coming to the table. If you are agitated, tense, or anxiety-ridden, your stomach will be in knots.

*Eat slowly* in a pleasant setting.

*If you are in the hospital, avoid eating in bed all the time.* Sit in a chair, go to the cafeteria with visitors, eat in the day room occasionally, or ask your doctor to give you a pass so you can go out to eat. Take a short walk between meals.

# Nausea

Nausea can be a problem at any stage of cancer treatment—from the initial work-up through the management phase, as it is a normal emotional reaction to anxiety and stress. It may be triggered by the diagnosis itself or by anticipation of treatment sessions, which are often preceded by a bout with nausea, either on the night before or on the morning of treatment.

Nausea can also be a temporary side effect of some treatment modalities, but it is usually or short duration. Sometimes it lasts longer and is followed by a period of queasiness. You can minimize it while it lasts by having confidence that it will pass and by trying these antidotes.

### Suggestions

*Suck on ice chips or anything frozen.*

*For early-morning or pre-meal nausea,* eat a dry bland food, like a cracker.

*Don't force yourself to eat* if you experience nausea for brief periods of time. Suck or bite on ice chips or something dry and hard until the feeling passes. Some people find sucking on lemon-flavored hard candy helpful.

*Make up for lost calories* when you feel more comfortable.

*If you become nauseated during or after treatment,* eat dry, bland, easy-to-digest foods several hours prior to treatment. This frequently reduces the degree of nausea. Stay away from heavy food or high-fat foods. (See Chapter 7 for more suggestions on eating.)

*If strong cooking aromas make you feel queasy or nauseous,* make sure that a venting fan is operating and try to remove yourself from the food preparation area. Eat your meals in a well-ventilated area free of odors. If no such place can be found, wait until the cooking odors have dissipated before you sit down to your meals.

*If the odor of the food itself makes you feel squeamish,* eliminate strong-smelling ones from your diet, and consciously select those that have little aroma and are unlikely to be cooked with garlic or other pungent seasonings. Try eating food chilled or frozen instead of warm or hot. Do not cover hot serving dishes because a burst of aroma arises when they are uncovered at the table.

*If these measures do not control the nausea,* try to arrange for someone else to cook or to go out for your meals. If you are the family cook, see Chapter 7 page 75 for additional suggestions.

*If you are in the hospital,* ask the nurse to remove the cover from your plate before bringing it into the room.

*Eat in a cool, conducive atmosphere* without upsetting distractions or odors.

*Keep liquids to a minimum,* as they create a feeling of fullness which aggravates queasiness or nausea.

*Eat and drink slowly.*

*Identify the foods you tolerate best* and make them your mainstay. Generally, low-fat foods (fruits, vegetables, sherbets), dry foods (pretzels, crackers, toast, dry cookies), and salty foods are usually well tolerated.

*Avoid* dishes that are fatty, greasy, or fried, overly sweet or heavily spiced, strongly flavored or odoriferous.

*Rest after eating,* to give your system a chance to digest the food. Lying flat immediately after eating a meal may start up the queasiness and discomfort, so elevate your head and shoulders above your chest.

*If vomiting relieves symptoms* of bloating, distention, or pain which accompany nausea, contact your physician.

*If nausea becomes constant or severe,* and your nutritional program is compromised for an extended period, your physician can prescribe medications to help alleviate it. Don't be shy about asking for one. Your doctor will not know your symptoms unless you tell him. Use members of your health care team as a resource, and discuss with them the problems you encounter between treatments. They are there to help you.

# Vomiting

If you feel nauseous, vomiting can readily be touched off. It may be an emotional response or a physical one caused by discomfort or bloating in the stomach or in the lower part of the gastrointestinal tract. Motion, activity, the consumption of food, and the smell, appearance, or even the thought of food can sometimes induce vomiting.

### Suggestions

*Eat frequent mini-meals* throughout the day to avoid feelings of fullness.

*Eat slowly* and chew your food well.

*Restrict fluids* to one hour before or after eating solid food.

*Eat dry food* like toast or crackers, and avoid sweets and fried or fatty food.

*Stay away from cooking odors.*

*Drink clear, cool beverages* like apple juice or flat ginger ale, or cola.

*Rest after eating,* but do not lie down flat for at least two hours.

*When you feel you are going to vomit,* lie down or rest, with your head and shoulders elevated, in a well-ventilated room free of unpleasant odors. Loosen any tight, constricting clothing, and put cool, damp cloths on your face and neck. Rinsing your mouth with mouthwash or cold water may also help allay the gagging or refluxing.

*If you do have periods of vomiting,* restrict all food and fluid until it subsides. Once it is under control, you can begin to drink small amounts of clear liquids—a few teaspoonfuls every ten to thirty minutes. (See Appendix F.) Gradually increase the amount. When you are sure the vomiting will not recur, progress to small amounts of soft, bland food and increase the portions by degrees until you are able to resume your normal diet.

*If you experience prolonged vomiting* and are unable to hold down any liquids for a period of two days, call your doctor. Dehydration is a serious consequence that must be combatted.

## Diarrhea and cramping

People who have a tendency to develop diarrhea or an upset stomach under stress or undue pressure will probably manifest those same symptoms temporarily during high-stress stages of cancer: the initial work-up, diagnosis, and treatments.

There are multiple causes for diarrhea during the treatment phase. It may be triggered by: (1) some drugs; (2) radiation or chemotherapy directed at the abdomen and/or chest; (3) sensitivities to certain foods; (4) a seriously compromised nutritional status or surgical removal of part of the GI tract; and (5) infections, particularly of the intestinal tract; and (6) other treatment modalities.

Prolonged, severe diarrhea puts you at risk of losing essential fluids and electrolytes. Long-term chronic diarrhea can bring about nutritional deficiencies because the rapid passage of food through the gastrointestinal tract does not allow sufficient time for absorption and utilization of nutrients.

### Suggestions

*Keep liquids to a minimum at mealtime, but drink between meals* to replace fluids and electrolytes, particularly sodium and potassium—minerals which can become depleted with prolonged diarrhea. Good between-meal liquids are clear broth and bouillon; flat ginger ale; and banana, peach, or apricot nectars.

*Eat mini-meals.*

*Drink all your liquids at a moderate temperature,* not hot or cold.

*Choose your solid foods carefully.* Stick with low-fiber items, like fish, chicken, well-ground meat, eggs, canned or well-cooked vegetables or fruits (without skins), ripe bananas, soft cereals, crackers, refined bread or flour products. Well-cooked mashed potatoes are usually well tolerated.

*Avoid* greasy, fatty, and fried foods, citrus juices, carbonated beverages, raw vegetables and fruits, and high-fiber foods like broccoli, corn, peas, lima beans, cauliflower, and natural grain breads, all of which are likely to stimulate bowel activity. Nuts, onions, garlic, and gas-forming vegetables (cauliflower, cabbage, beans, and broccoli) also seem to be bowel irritants.

*If you have persistent diarrhea,* rest or keep activity to a minimum after meals to decrease the intestinal activity and peristalsis which control the rate of food passage.

*If you have severe diarrhea,* restrict your intake to clear, room-temperature liquids like broth, flat ginger ale, or apple juice for a day (see Appendix A). This will replace lost fluids and allow the bowel to rest. Try to estimate your fluid losses and do your best to replace them. When the diarrhea is controlled, you can try other liquids and soft, bland, low-fiber food. If the situation remains stable, gradually return to a more normal diet and make up your nutritional losses.

*If you have occasional cramps or gas pain,* avoid beer, highly carbonated soft drinks, beans, cabbage, broccoli, cauliflower, and onions. Sweet or highly spiced foods may also produce gas symptoms. Chew your food with your mouth closed, and be careful not to gulp or swallow air while eating because it will increase the cramps and pressure.

*If cramping continues* or is accompanied by vomiting, consult your doctor.

*If diarrhea is uncontrollable or persistent,* your physician can order medication to ease it.

*If diarrhea is bloody,* notify your doctor immediately.

# Constipation

Constipation can be caused by some drugs, particularly pain medications or certain chemotherapeutic agents. It can also result from the type of diet you consume. Liquid, soft, or low-fiber diets can cause constipation if they are followed for a considerable period of time.

### Suggestions

*Six to eight glasses of fluid a day* and an increased intake of high-fiber foods like whole grain cereals and breads, bran, dried fruit, and raw fruits and vegetables should help. See Appendix E for foods that are high in fiber.

*Take a walk* or exercise after eating.

*If these measures do not succeed,* check with your doctor or nurse. Do not use laxatives without your physician's permission.

# Mouth sores (stomatitis or mucositis)

Sores resulting from certain types of treatment can occur in the mouth and occasionally further down the GI tract. The accompanying discomfort can limit food intake.

## Suggestions

*Take scrupulous care of your mouth and gums* to help prevent infections. Use a soft-bristled toothbrush, and don't brush too hard. Your pharmacy sells oral swabs which can also be used to clean your teeth.

*Do not use commercial mouthwashes* with a high salt or alcohol content. You can make your own by mixing one teaspoon of bicarbonate of soda (baking soda) with one cupful of warm water. Keep this rinse in your mouth for about one minute.

*If you have mouth sores,* avoid highly acidic foods like tomatoes, oranges, and grapefruit, which may sting your mouth, and salty or spicy food, which may cause a burning sensation. Cigarettes and alcohol are also irritants.

*If your mouth becomes very tender and irritated,* stick to soft, unseasoned foods or a liquid diet. Ask your physician if he advocates a medication.

# Ostomy

Ostomies are surgically constructed openings, usually in the lower abdomen, that allow the excretion of wastes when the usual routes are damaged or removed.

An urostomy is used to collect liquid wastes after removal or surgical diversion of the bladder or ureturs. A colostomy is used after the rectum or part of the colon has been removed and an ileostomy is used after the removal of the entire colon.

Immediately after surgery, for a colostomy or ileostomy, you may be given a low-residue diet to permit your bowel to rest and adjust to the new elimination routine. However, once adjusted, ostomates can live a normal life in every way, including the way they eat. Good nutrition remains vital after an ostomy; and the proper selection of foods will help avoid potential problems such as blockages, diarrhea, gas, or odor.

Following an urostomy you will probably be instructed to drink lots of plain liquids to reduce the risk of infection or the formation of kidney stones.

## Suggestions for all ostomies

*Contact your local chapter of the United Ostomy Association* (See Chapter 9). It is an excellent support group that has information to help you adjust to almost any routine situation.

*If you need extra help,* ask for a referral to an enterostomal therapist, a specially trained and certified professional who can help you make the necessary adjustments in your living pattern. If one is not available in your area, perhaps your local chapter of the United Ostomy Association can bring one to your area to consult with the group. (Contact: International Association for Enterostomal Therapy, 505 North Tustin Avenue, Suite 282, Santa Ana, CA 92705.)

## Suggestions for colostomy and ileostomy

*To avoid blockages,* be careful about eating high-fiber foods like celery or vegetables with kernels or seeds. Add new foods to your diet one at a time so you can evaluate their effects and identify undesirable reactions. Stay away from any foods that have caused problems in the past.

*To avoid diarrhea,* be careful about eating spicy food, raw fruits and vegetables, fruit juices, and beer, and avoid any foods that caused diarrhea in the past.

*If diarrhea occurs,* return to a low-residue diet. Drink small amounts of tea or boiled milk, and contact your doctor if it is severe or prolonged.

*To avoid gas,* always chew your food with your mouth closed. Don't skip meals. Avoid carbonated beverages. Don't chew gum. Check your irrigation schedule.

*Odor is seldom a problem* for ostomates. However, if you do have a problem, avoid gas producing foods like onions, beans, cabbage, and eggs; and use odorproof, disposable appliances or a commercial deodorizing liquid or tablet. If odor does become detectable, your doctor can prescribe an oral medication to combat it.

## Weight gain

While some people react to stress or anxiety by losing their appetites, others respond by overeating. Indeed, eating for solace is a fairly common phenomenon in the general population. Stimulation of appetite and subsequent weight gain can be a side-effect of some drugs used in cancer therapy, such as steroids.

*If you have gained an excessive amount of weight*, check with your doctor before starting a reducing program. He or she may feel that you should complete treatment before attempting to lose weight.

*Do not go on a nutritionally unbalanced fad diet.* This is not the time to place any unnecessary stress on your body. If your doctor approves, select a well-balanced calorie-reduction diet, or ask your doctor to refer you to a dietitian.

## Water retention

Edema, or water retention, occurs because the tissues hold excess fluid. It can result from the cancer itself or be induced as a side effect of some treatments, malnutrition, or drugs. When edema occurs, discuss the cause and treatment with your physician. If he or she prescribes a low-sodium diet, the following suggestions should help.

### Suggestions

*Decrease your salt intake* by eliminating table salt and reducing the amount of salt you use in cooking.

*Read food package labels.* Try to buy brands that do not mention salt, sodium, MSG, baking soda, or baking powder high on the list of ingredients.

*Refer to Appendix B* for a moderately low sodium diet plan.

*If you need a strictly controlled sodium diet*, ask your doctor to refer you to a dietitian, and check Chapter 9 for relevent books and pamphlets.

## Lactose intolerance

Lactose is the sugar found in milk and milk products. A lactose intolerance signals that your body does not manufacture sufficient lactase, the enzyme needed to digest lactose. When lactose is not broken down in the intestinal tract by this enzyme, undigested lactose remains in the intestine, which then draws in large amounts of water in an effort to dilute it. In addition, bacteria present in the GI tract ferment the undigested lactose; and the result of the increased fluid volume and gaseous fermentation is cramps, increased motility, distention, and diarrhea. Several treatment programs can produce a lactose intolerance. The degree varies from one person to another, depending on the amount of decrease in lactase activity. You must monitor your intake of milk and dairy products to find out how much lactose you can consume without becoming symptomatic.

Suggestions

*Try yogurt, buttermilk, and processed cheeses.* Sometimes these foods can be tolerated.

*Use lactose-free dairy substitutes* like Mocha-Mix, Dairy Rich, imitation sour cream, and non-dairy whipped toppings like Cool Whip.

*If you are completely lactase deficient or severely intolerant,* you will need to read the labels of all prepared foods that might contain milk or a milk product. Read carefully: lactose is also frequently used as a sweetening agent in foods.

*Eliminate or evaluate all milk and milk-based items* in your diet. Any products containing whey, casein, or nonfat milk solids should be avoided or tested in small amounts to gauge their effects (see Appendix C).

*Check medications,* since lactose is also used as a filler in some tablet-type medications.

*Read labels,* lactose is often used as a sweetening agent in foods.

*If you wish to use milk as a beverage in cooking,* add Lact-Aid, a commercial lactase enzyme which hydrolyzes the lactose in milk prior to use. Lactase taken by mouth is ineffective. It must come in direct contact with the milk sugar for a specified amount of time to perform its function. Be sure to read product instructions before using any commercial lactase enzyme. If your pharmacy does not carry Lact-Aid, contact the manufacturer: Sugar Lo Company, P.O. Box 111, 600 Fire Road, Pleasantville, NJ 08232 (800) 257-8650.

*If you find you are unable to eat adequate amounts of milk products,* ask your physician about alternate sources of calcium.

*Refer to Appendix C* for a lactose-free diet.

# Pain

Cancer is not always accompanied by pain. Many new techniques for controlling pain have been developed in the last few years. If pain does occur, there are several approaches to relieve or reduce it: medications, operations on nerves, nerve blocks, and techniques such as relaxation, distraction, biofeedback, acupuncture, or hypnosis.

Oncologists, anesthesiologists, and other doctors or nurses may be pain specialists. Chapter 9 gives a list of sources that can provide the names of consultants or pain programs in your locality and a partial list of pain centers in the United States.

Your physician may suggest a center that he is familiar with, or your local American Cancer Society can put you in contact with a nearby pain program.

### Suggestions

*Pain medication should be taken about an hour before mealtime* for maximum effectiveness when you sit down to eat.

*Some find that a cocktail, beer, or wine* before meals not only stimulates the appetite but also acts as a mild pain killer. Check with your doctor before drinking alcohol to make sure it does not interfere with any of your medications.

*You may want to investigate* some of the new alternative treatments, like biofeedback, that have enabled many to control or alleviate pain.


## What to do when you simply cannot eat enough

Fortunately, there are other simple, easy ways to obtain adequate nutrition if all your efforts to eat frequent, small, nutrient-dense meals fail, and you cannot meet your nutritional requirements. The most effective method for most people is tube feeding. Unfortunately, many people are frightened by the idea of being fed through a tube. For them, the very thought of tube feeding conjures up an image from some late-night horror movie of a hapless victim of a mad scientist who is being kept alive by means of grotesque tubes. This mental picture has kept many people from even discussing the possibility of tube feeding with their doctors.

The truth of the matter is that thousands of people are taking advantage of this simple, efficient method because it is so easy and eliminates the pressures of eating unwanted meals. The tubes are very thin and soft, like a piece of finely cooked spaghetti, and are very well tolerated. The nutritionally complete liquid formulas available for tube feeding can be used to fill all your nutrient needs, leaving you free to eat just those foods that appeal to you, or not to "eat" at all.

You can choose from a variety of inexpensive tubes, containers, and very small feeding delivery systems that allow you to feed yourself with a minimum of effort.

## Tube feeding

Tube feeding allows you maximum freedom and flexibility; you decide when and where you want to eat. Some people prefer to take their feedings during the day while they are sitting around relaxing or watching television. Others who work or go to school prefer to feed themselves in the evening or at night.

If you feel you might benefit from this type of feeding technique, discuss it with your physician.

### Liquid formulas

You can make your own formula (see Appendix I) or choose from the variety of commercial products available. Appendix G lists the names and addresses of companies that manufacture these products. If the formula suggested by your medical care team is not available in your local pharmacy, ask the pharmacist to stock it or write directly to the manufacturer. These formulas are designed to be used as total meal replacements, nutritional supplements, or calorie boosters. The products mentioned as total meal replacements are nutritionally complete—that is they provide adequate protein, energy, vitamins, minerals, and trace elements if consumed in a sufficient quantity (a volume equivalent to your daily needs, usually about 2000 calories).

*For a fine-bore feeding tube,* you need a well-homogenized formula that will not clog the thin, flexible tube.

*Some products have special nutritional characteristics,* so it is important to be aware of any specific medical or nutritional requirements you may have and select the product that will meet your individual needs.

*Compare prices and content,* so you do not pay for special features you do not need.

*If you have no special requirements and need a supplement* to boost calories or as a replacement for beverages containing little or no nutrition, the following products are appropriate: Carnation Instant

**TABLE 3-1  SPECIAL FEATURES OF LIQUID FORMULAS**

| Product | High calorie | Non sweetened | Low sodium | Low potassium | Lactose free | Low fat |
|---|---|---|---|---|---|---|
| Ensure | | | | | X | |
| Ensure Plus | X | | | | X | |
| Isocal | | X | | | X | |
| Isocal HCN | X | | X | X | X | |
| Magnacal | X | | | X | X | |
| Osmolite | | X | | X | X | MCT oil = $\frac{1}{2}$ fat source |
| Precision HN | | | | | X | X |
| Precision Isotonic | | | | | X | |
| Precision LR | | | | X | X | X |
| Renu | | | | | X | |
| Travasorb MCT | X | | X | | X | MCT oil = primary fat source |
| Travasorb liquid | | | | | X | |
| Sustacal | | | | | X | |
| Sustacal HC | X | | | | X | |

See Appendix G for manufacturers names and addresses.

Breakfast, or Nutriment, which can be purchased in a supermarket or Ensure, Meritene Liquid or Powder, Travsorb Liquid, Sustacal Powder or Liquid, Sustagen Powder, which can be purchased at your pharmacy. Unless otherwise specified these products contain milk. If you have a lactose intolerance or suspect one, test the product first or select a lactose-free product.

*If you need a lactose-free, low-residue supplement or meal replacement,* select one of the products listed in Table 3-1. The special characteristics of each product is listed. All products in this group contain at least thirty calories per ounce or one calorie per milliliter.

*If you need a simple tube feeding as a meal replacement and have no special requirements,* you can use any of the products listed in Table 3-1, the homemade tube feeding in Appendix I, or any of the following products: Compleat-B, Compleat Modified (lactose free), Formula-2, or Vitaneed (lactose free). This latter group of products contains regular foods blended together to provide a wholesome, well-balanced complete diet which can easily pass through a tube. Be sure to do some price comparisons. Many of the products listed in Appendix G may be cheaper and will also meet your needs.

*If you are unable to digest or absorb food in your intestinal tract in a normal fashion,* you will need professional help in selecting a formula. Although there are products that can be taken by mouth, they are not especially tasty and are usually reserved for tube feeding. Ask your doctor or dietitian which product would be best for you.

*If you have an eating problem that is going to necessitate prolonged tube feeding,* you may want to ask your doctor to help you evaluate techniques such as feeding gastrostomy.

*If you need help at home,* there are now commercial companies that will work with your medical team to provide supplies and equipment for home use. This service is often covered by insurance. Ask your medical team, particularly the social worker, for the names of national and local companies

*Check your insurance coverage.* Some companies will reimburse you for tube feeding if you have a physician's prescription.

## Physical limitations

If you have a physical limitation or disability that interferes with your ability to eat—for example, difficulty using your hand or arm—ask your doctor to refer you to a physical or occupational therapist. These medical professionals can help you locate the numerous specially designed devices to assist people with physical limitations.

# 4

## CANCER OF THE GASTRO-
## INTESTINAL TRACT

The cells that make up the gastrointestinal tract (GI tract) are replaced or "turned over" more rapidly than many of the other cells in your body. For this reason they are particularly sensitive to cancer therapy which, as you learned in Chapter 1, is aimed at rapidly growing cells.

Any disturbance in the GI tract, whether from cancer itself or its treatment can have a potentially adverse effect on your nutritional status.

Cancer in the various parts of the GI tract are discussed in this chapter. Hopefully the suggestions offered here, as well as those offered in Chapters 1 and 3, will help you deal with any problems that might arise.

### Cancer of the mouth, tongue, and throat

Surgery in the oral cavity or in the throat can result in obvious mechanical problems in chewing and swallowing. Radiation in this area can also result in a variety of effects which can affect your food intake and consequently your nutritional status. Radiation can cause a loss of taste known as *mouth blindness* or a decrease in salivary secretions, which manifests itself as a dry mouth. It can also affect the jaws and teeth, thereby limiting your ability to chew and swallow naturally. Some people find that their throats become irritated and sore, and swallowing becomes difficult. Fortunately, these symptoms usually subside shortly after the immediate exposure to radiation, but it is important to maintain fluid intake even during these acute periods.

A loss of appetite resulting from emotional or physical stress, coupled with mechanical problems, can put you at risk of becoming severely malnourished if you don't systematically compensate nutritionally. Fortunately there are a number of ways you can enhance your appetite and your enjoyment of food under these circumstances.

If you have trouble developing an appropriate feeding plan, consult your physician, your clinical dietitian, or your nutritionist. They can help you structure a plan and a feeding schedule to meet your individual needs.

## Suggestions

*Plan menus that smell good and are pleasing to the eye.* Make sure that the surroundings are pleasant and the food is appetizingly presented when you sit down to eat. If food seems dry or hard to chew, include moist or liquid foods in your menus (see Chapter 6 and recipe chapters for suggestions).

*If salivary secretions are decreased,* eat soft, moist food; use extra sauces, and drink liquids with food (see Chapter 3 and recipe chapters and Appendix H for additional ideas).

*If your food is tasteless and you do not have a sore mouth and throat,* try eating salty food or seasoning your food generously with your favorite spices and condiments. Concentrate on eating foods with distinctive textures, such as rice pudding with raisins, fruits with crunchy peanut butter, chicken or shrimp salads, barely cooked vegetables, Chinese food, or casseroles topped with nuts or crunchy toppings, so you can feel the food in your mouth.

*If your mouth and/or throat are sore,* stick to soft, bland food that is easy to chew and swallow. Incorporate calorically dense beverages like milkshakes, eggnogs, and liquid-complete nutritional formulas (Appendix G) until you can return to a normal diet.

*If a surgical procedure on the mouth, tongue, or neck seriously impairs chewing or swallowing,* tube feeding may be required. The tube bypasses the affected area and carries liquid food directly to your stomach. This is an easy, effective way to get nourishment when there is a mechanical problem affecting your ability to eat properly.

For tube feedings, you can use a blenderized version of the same foods your family eats, as long as it is nutritionally balanced (see Appendix I), or use a commercial product (see Appendix G). At the present time, there are over thirty different liquid products available which provide all the nutrients needed for a good diet. If you require a special diet, for example, a low-lactose, low-fat, or low-salt diet, an appropriate formula can be prescribed for you by a dietitian. All these products are not exactly the same so it is a good idea to check with your physician or dietitian before selecting one. See page 36 for additional information and suggestions on tube feeding.

# Esophagus

When the esophagus is involved, you may find that you are unable to swallow or that swallowed food will not stay down because it cannot pass a stricture or closure caused by the tumor or by tissue swelling. If you experience this type of problem, you will probably find that the esophagus begins to open up with treatment, enabling you to gradually return to a normal diet. However, until the esophagus is fully opened, you may not be able to maintain adequate nutritional intake by conventional means. Under these circumstances, your physician may recommend a liquid diet, tube feeding, or intravenous feeding to prevent dehydration or malnourishment during this period. If major nutritional problems develop following surgery, these are best handled by trained medical professionals.

# Stomach

Maintaining adequate calorie intake is a major nutritional problem for anyone who has had stomach surgery or is undergoing some type of treatment in the stomach area. It is easy to incur a calorie deficit because the stomach's capacity to do its job is diminished, and there is a tendency to feel full after eating only a small amount of food.

The stomach is a reservoir where food is held for mixing and homogenizing. Surgery in the stomach can hinder the digestion of some foods, causing them to flow undigested or too rapidly into the intestine. Abdominal distention and discomfort accompanied by dizziness, weakness, flushing, or sweating can result. These sensations may be followed by nausea, vomiting, or diarrhea.

### Suggestions

*To decrease or eliminate these side effects;* try not to overwhelm your system. Eat slowly and chew your food thoroughly. If you can tolerate it, eat frequent, small meals, consisting largely of protein with some fat and complex carbohydrates. Don't drink fluids with your meals since they tend to propel foods through the stomach into the intestine. Avoid highly osmotic foods (foods containing a predominance of simple sugars or carbohydrates), which will cause your system to pull extra fluids into the GI tract to dilute them. You may find it helpful to lie down following meals.

*Keep your spirits up.* These effects usually subside with time, so be patient.

*Keep vitamin and mineral intake adequate.* Two important functions of the stomach are related to the production of iron and the utilization of vitamin B12. Your doctor will be monitoring your iron and B12 levels to guard against a deficiency of either of these two essential nutrients.

## Small and large intestine

Some people find that radiation or chemotherapy in the intestinal tract—the small and large bowel—has a marked effect on their ability to handle food. The lining of the intestinal tract is extremely sensitive because new cells are constantly replacing old ones at a rapid rate. Treatments that are designed to kill fast-growing cancer cells can also affect normal cells in the intestinal lining and alter its function. In most cases, symptoms, like diarrhea or nausea, will disappear within a short period following the termination of the treatment program. However, some people may experience prolonged or delayed effects. Chapter 3 gives specific instructions for handling symptoms you may develop.

When there has been a partial or significant removal of the intestines, you may need to pay close attention to your nutritional status. It is essential to work closely with the medical team and the dietary staff, because dietary management in this instance involves very complex considerations. It is not advisable to try to handle these problems on your own.

## Pancreas

A decrease in pancreatic enzyme can cause you to have severe digestive problems which can result in nutritional deficiencies. The nutritional implications are complicated and best handled by a trained nutritional-medical team. A high carbohydrate diet is usually ordered, as carbohydrates are easily digested and absorbed without good pancreatic function; and dietary fat is often minimized because it causes much of the gas, rumbling, bloating, and diarrhea that may occur.

To provide fat which your body requires for basic functions, medium chain triglycerides (MCT) are often recommended because they are well absorbed without pancreatic action. These fats are available commercially as MCT oil and in a premixed form in complete nutritional feedings (see Appendix G). If you can tolerate the fat contained in chocolate syrup, a small amount disguises the taste of the oil quite well. If your physician prescribes MCT oil or a product that contains it, be careful not to take a large dose all at once because an excess can cause discomfort or diarrhea. Consult your physician if diarrhea becomes chronic.

# 5

## NUTRITION FOR

## CHILDREN WITH CANCER

Even when they are feeling well, there are some children who pride themselves on being finicky eaters. And, their parents, who realize how important good nutrition is for growth and development, are caught in a seemingly endless struggle to get their reluctant offspring to eat correctly. The parents of a sick child often are faced with a finicky eater. Sometimes it may be because he or she is just feeling ornery, but most of the time there are a multitude of good reasons for the child's lack of interest in food.

All of us—children and adults—experience a loss of appetite when we are feeling ill. If we have a short illness, the body can recover quickly to its pre-illness state of well being. However, if the illness is prolonged, as with a chronic illness like cancer, your body may begin to suffer from the ill effects of malnutrition if appropriate steps are not taken on an ongoing basis. In addition, many of us experience responses to stress that are manifested in ways that affect our ability or desire to eat.

## How cancer can affect a child's nutritional status

Cancer is a long-term illness that can greatly affect a child's appetite and tolerance for food in many ways. First, the emotional trauma associated with such a serious illness can have a profound effect on the child and can impact his or her appetite or ability to eat. Loss of appetite, heartburn, nausea, vomiting, diarrhea—all can be symptoms of emotional stress.

Surgery on any part of the gastrointestinal tract can be a source of potential nutritional problems. Some of the treatments used for cancer can have one or more side effects that can influence the child's desire or ability to eat. Any one of the following effects can significantly impact a child's nutritional status: loss of appetite, feeling of fullness, heartburn, nausea, vomiting, cramping, diarrhea, constipation, inability to absorb nutrients, "dry mouth," sore mouth or throat, loss of taste sensation, weakness, or pain. These effects will reduce food intake to varying degrees.

Not all children have side effects from therapy but, unfortunately, a certain number do. Many of these children suffer from a combination of emotional and physical symptoms. Because of a child's small size and need for adequate nutrients to support growth, if immediate steps are not taken, these symptoms can rapidly lead to a weight loss and a deteriorating nutritional state.

## Nutrition program for children with cancer

The basic principles underlying the nutrition program for a child with cancer is similar to the program for any child: It must include the right balance of nutrients needed to promote continuous growth and development. Please note that a stable weight is not always a reliable indicator of nutritional status in children. Children should be gaining weight gradually as they grow. Therefore, a nutrition program for a child with cancer must not only include enough calories to avoid weight loss and promote weight gain, but also enough calories to cope with the additional stress of the disease and its treatment. By doing this, you will be doing the best you can to ensure constant growth.

A well-nourished child should be well within the normal limits of height and weight for age as illustrated in Appendix J. For most children, following recommendations in Table 5-1 will provide for an adequate intake of protein and calories. If your child is losing weight or failing to grow or gain adequate weight for his or her age, these levels may have to be raised.

To make sure your child is getting the right balance of all nutrients—protein, fat, carbohydrate, vitamins, and minerals—needed for optimum body functioning, provide a diet made up

**TABLE 5-1   CHILDREN'S REQUIREMENTS**

| | Age in Years | | | | |
|---|---|---|---|---|---|
| | 1 | 1–3 | 4–6 | 7–10 | 11–14 |
| Calories lb/day | 50 | 45 | 40 | 36 | 23 |
| Protein gm/lb/day | 1 | 0.8 | 0.7 | 0.54 | 0.45 |

EXAMPLE: To calculate the appropriate amounts of calories and protein for a 5-year-old child weighing 35 pounds, multiply: 35 pounds × 40 calories/pound = 1400 calories/day

35 pounds × 0.7 grams protein/pound = 24.5 gm protein/day

from a variety of foods included in the basic four food groups. You may want to review the information on food and nutrition given in Chapter 2 and refer to Table 2-1. Table 2-1 gives recommendations on the specific number of servings from the basic four food groups needed at various age levels to promote good health.

If your child is having difficulty eating a balanced diet, you may want to ask your doctor about a vitamin and mineral supplement. However, there is absolutely no validity to claims that megadoses of vitamins are helpful in the treatment of cancer. In fact, some vitamins can interfere with certain cancer therapies. So, to be on the safe side, check with your child's physician before starting any vitamin or mineral supplement. For that matter, it is a good idea to always check with the physician in charge of your child's care before giving any over-the-counter medication or medication prescribed by another doctor because there is always a possibility of a drug interaction.

The recommendations given here are general recommendations. The needs of children can vary with age, activity level, and nutritional status, so the best approach is to consult with the medical team in charge of your child's care to determine the exact nutritional goals for your child. A close, cooperative, ongoing relationship between you and the medical team is essential for the well-being of your child. Any time your child shows signs of losing grounds nutritionally, seek professional help from the physician or dietition. It is far easier to maintain weight than to regain lost weight, so don't be shy. Even if you don't get an immediate response, keep right on asking for the help you need. Medical professionals can sometimes become preoccupied with the other details of a specific treatment program and need to be reminded about the nutritional needs of their patients. Also remember doctors cannot be expected to be experts in everything and most have very little experience in the field of nutrition. If you think it is needed, ask for a referral to a dietitian or nutritionist who has the background and training to help you deal with nutrition and dietary problems.

## Your role as a parent

Don't ever be reluctant to ask questions about your child's treatment or disease. This is a confusing and stressful time for you, your child, and the rest of your family. You may need to ask and re-ask for explanations about your child's disease and the treatment program until it is clear to you. If there are things you don't understand, be persistent and keep seeking the help you need. You, as a parent, are being called on to make many decisions concerning your child and you need to be well informed.

Your doctor and the medical team caring for your child are the best sources of information, but they are not available 24 hours a day. Seek additional sources of *reliable* information. Chapter 9 contains a listing of some good sources of information and at the end of this chapter there is a list of publications geared specifically to children with cancer and their families.

At the present time no one knows exactly why children get cancer. And as unfair as it is, it is unfortunately true that some children develop terrible diseases. But, as far as anyone knows, there was nothing you or your child did to cause this disease, so don't ever feel guilty. Use your energy in a positive way. Do your best to be supportive of your child during this very difficult time and cooperate with the medical team that is trying to control or eradicate your child's cancer.

Most parents find a gentle, honest approach to their child works best. Create an open, ongoing communication and let your child know that you understand and share his or her feelings and fears. Do your best to comfort and reassure the child who suffers side effects from cancer or its treatment. Explain that although it is very difficult right now, side effects are usually temporary and the treatments, although very difficult, are designed to help him get better.

And, if there is only one idea you take away from this chapter let it be this: Don't try to "go it alone." Get all the help and support you can for you and your child. Don't be embarrassed to ask for emotional support from outside sources: psychiatrist, psychologist, social workers, chaplains, friends, family, other parents, and cancer support groups. It would be very unusual if you were able to remain always calm, cool, and collected during such a difficult time in your life. Chances are you will be better equipped to help your child if you yourself get some help and support in dealing with the overwhelming problems that can beset the family of a child with cancer.

## Feeding problems and what you can do

First of all, try to relax and maintain a calm, positive approach to food and nutrition. Encourage your child to stock up on calories and nutrients during periods when he or she is feeling well and don't try to force your child to eat a normal diet on bad days. The suggestions outlined below, as well as those in Chapter 3 and other sections of the book, should help. But before you start to develop a nutrition program for your child, there are a few overriding principles concerning children and food and nutrition you should know about.

1. Children's appetites seem to change constantly and they often need to eat more frequently than adults. They often are not hungry at the usual mealtimes and are starving at other times throughout the day.
2. Young children do not require as much food as adults. One tablespoon of each type of food—meat or meat substitute, dairy products, fruits, vegetables, grain products—at each meal for each year of life is generally sufficient. For example, a three-year old needs three tablespoons of each type of food.
3. What a child eats is more important than how much is eaten or when it is eaten. Small servings of nutritious foods eaten throughout the day may be more helpful than the traditional three meals a day.
4. A child's appetite can vary, depending on the level of activity and whether or not the child is in an active growth period.
5. Children are notoriously fussy eaters whether they are sick or well. Children often use food as a tool to get attention or to get their own way. This is particularly difficult for the parents of a sick child who must determine whether or not it is the illness that is causing the problem.

*Suggestions*

*Relax and try to make mealtimes a happy experience.* Don't nag a child who feels too ill to eat.

*Make the mealtime surroundings as pleasant as possible.* Try rotating the surroundings—a box lunch in front of the TV, an outdoor picnic, lunch at a favorite restaurant.

*Prepare meals with eye appeal.* Use colorful garnishes and bite size portions with fancy toothpicks. Serve food on fun dishes. Set the table with pretty placemats, fancy napkins, or a silly centerpiece. Serve drinks with a trick straw or a sandwich in a toy truck.

*Remember children eat at varying rates.* Don't try to hurry up the slow poke, and let a fast eater leave the table when he or she is finished.

*Involvement often stimulates interest in food.* Let your child help you do the grocery shopping or help you with the food preparation. Many children will eat what they themselves prepare. Encourage your child to make nutritious snacks or fun desserts.

*Don't use mealtimes for a nutrition lesson.* And don't withhold dessert when your child doesn't eat the main part of the meal. Wait until after the meal to explain why good food is important.

*Add extra nutrition to foods.* Add nonfat dry milk powder or eggs to dishes like puddings, milkshakes, and casseroles. Spread peanut butter or cheese on fruit slices. Add bite-size pieces of meat and vegetables to soups. Use high protein milk (see page 67) whenever a recipe calls for milk.

*Serve essential nutrients in a high-powered form children like.* Milkshakes made with commercial nutritional supplements (see Appendix G) can be excellent sources of nutrition for children. Nutritional supplements in the form of pudding are also available.

*Respect your child's food dislikes.* There are so many nutritious foods available to choose from, why have a confrontation? If your child refuses to eat meat, substitute cheese, eggs, peanut butter, or tuna fish—all favorites with kids. If cooked vegetables pose a problem, substitute raw fruit and vegetables cut in bite size pieces or served with a yummy dip.

Some cancer treatments can effect taste sensations so foods previously eaten may be rejected and those previously scorned may turn out to be favorites! Don't despair, just be flexible, smile, and try the food again later.

*Don't expect your child to eat if he or she is receiving intensive anticancer therapy that causes side effects.* Wait until the child is feeling better to encourage a normal diet. Let your child eat whenever he or she wants and whatever foods appeal at that particular time.

*If nausea and vomiting are problems,* withhold all liquid and solid food until the vomiting is controlled. Make your child comfortable, elevate the head slightly, and make sure that the room is well-ventilated. Loosen any constricting clothing. Wipe the child's face with a cool, damp cloth and make sure that any soiled bed linen is removed immediately.

*To avoid any chance of aspiration, never force solid food on a child who has been vomiting.*

*Once vomiting is controlled* encourage your child to drink liquids: start with one teaspoon every ten minutes, gradually increasing to one tablespoon every 20 minutes and then two tablespoons every 30 minutes. Liquids such as broth or boullion, Jell-O, carbonated drinks (some like them flat), Kool-Aid, popsicles, Gatorade, and fruit ice are usually well tolerated. If these are tolerated well and symptoms have subsided, offer the child soft, low-fat, easy-to-digest foods that don't have strong aromas. Foods at room temperature or cold may be better tolerated than hot ones. Good choices are soda crackers, unbuttered toast, baked potatoes, rice, and skinned chicken breasts. Avoid milk products. Encourage small frequent feedings in a well ventilated room. Avoid serving liquids with solid foods.

*If vomiting is a common problem,* ask your child's physician to prescribe a medication to help control it.

*Always contact your doctor* if your child begins to vomit for no apparent reason or if vomiting persists or is unusually severe.

*If diarrhea is a problem,* give your child a diet that eliminates raw fruits and vegetables, milk, high fat and fried foods and whole grain products (see low-residue diet, Appendix F). If this doesn't control it, ask your doctor for medication. Also check to see if your child might have a lactose intolerance which could be causing the diarrhea.

Small frequent feedings and lying down immediately after meals will often help control diarrhea.

*If diarrhea follows the treatment,* start the child on a clear liquid diet and gradually advance to full liquids followed by a soft, low-residue diet that is also low in fat (see Appendix F). Very hot or cold foods may be irritating. Do not serve liquids with solid foods.

*If diarrhea persists* for more than two days, is unusually severe, or is bloody, contact your child's physician at once.

*If chewing or swallowing is a problem,* try a soft diet and cut all foods into small, bite-size pieces. Scrambled eggs, cooked cereals, creamed soups, puddings, ice cream, milkshakes, eggnogs, flaked fish, mashed potatoes, pasta, stewed fruits, cooked vegetables, yogurt, and cottage cheese are all good choices. Serve foods with sauces and gravies.

*If your child has mouth sores,* check with your doctor or dentist to get advice on special mouth care. Make sure your child rinses his or her mouth frequently. Try straws for liquids, and serve soft foods cut in tiny pieces or in sauces. You may even want to puree foods. Ice cream, pudding, milkshakes, bananas, cottage cheese, canned pears and peaches, yogurt, macaroni and cheese, souffles, and quiches are all easy to handle. Avoid acidic foods (tomatoes, oranges, grapefruit), spicy foods, very salty foods, or foods that have a rough texture like toast or raw fruit and vegetables.

## Some nutritious snacks for children

Cream cheese on date nut bread, fruit slices or crackers
Melted cheese on toast
Granola
Cheese and crackers
Milkshakes
Sandwiches with meat
Peanut butter on celery sticks
Fruit slices and crackers
High calorie, milk-based desserts
Cheesecake
Bread products with extra jelly and butter
Cakes and cookies made with whole grains
Fruits, nuts, wheatgerm
Cereal with milk
Creamed soups
Buttered popcorn
Pizza

Dips made with cream cheese or sour cream
Peanuts and other nuts
Raw vegetables with dips
Fruit slices with yogurt dips
Fresh and canned fruit with high-caloric topping
Dried fruits like raisins, prunes, or apricots
Deviled eggs
Hardboiled eggs
Pudding and custards
Yogurt
Ice cream with syrup for extra calories
Chocolate milk
High protein milk (see page 67)
Eggnog
Cottage cheese
Hamburgers
Any cheeses

See Chapter 6 for ideas for adding calories and protein foods.

## Special reading material for children with cancer and their families

*Hospital Days—Treatment Ways.* J. Warmbier; E. Vassy. 1978. Free
A hematology-oncology coloring book designed to familiarize pediatric cancer patients with some of the hospital diagnostic and treatment procedures that they may observe or experience. Parents are encouraged to explore the book with their child, allowing the child to express his feelings about the pictures. To assist parents in this interaction, a guide to the illustrations is provided.

» *National Cancer Institute Office of Cancer Communications*
*Bldg. 31, Room 10A18*
*9000 Rockville Pike*
*Bethesda, MD 20205*

*A Story About Leukemia to Color.* P. S. Tharp; J. A. Dobos. 1978. Mailing charges only

A coloring book designed to help pediatric patients explore their feelings and fears about leukemia.

» *Cancer Center of University Hospitals*
*At-Home Rehabilitation Program*
*2074 Abington Rd.*
*Cleveland, OH 44106*
*(216) 444-3783*

*There Is a Rainbow Behind Every Dark Cloud.* 1978. $6.95

A book designed to help the child deal with his fears. The emphasis is on living in the present and healing oneself by maintaining a positive attitude. It is written and illustrated by children for children who have leukemia or other life-threatening illnesses. It discusses the medical and emotional experiences these patients will encounter.

» *Center for Attitudinal Healing*
*19 Main St.*
*Tiburon, CA 94920*
*(415) 435-5022*

*You and Leukemia: A Day at a Time.* L. S. Baker, Rev. 1978. $7.95

A handbook on childhood leukemia, addressed to children over nine or ten years of age. It covers the pertinent facts about this kind of cancer: symptoms, diagnosis and treatment, and complications. Chemotherapy drugs are listed individually and their possible side effects detailed. Illustrations reinforce the text throughout and blank pages are provided for patients to record their own treatment programs or to draw pictures.

» *W. B. Saunders Co.*
*W. Washington Sq.*
*Philadelphia, PA 19105*
*(215) 574-4700*

*What Happened to You Happened to Me.* J. A. Kjosness; L. A. Rudolph, eds. 1980. Free

A booklet illustrated and written by young people with cancer to help other childhood cancer patients with worries and concerns they may have. Twelve separate sections deal with the experiences that young people with cancer have in common and offer suggestions for coping with these.

» *The Children's Orthopedic Hospital and Medical Center*
*Division of Pediatric Hematology/Oncology*
*4800 Sand Point Way, N.E.*
*P.O. Box C5371*
*Seattle, WA 98105*
*(206) 634-5427*

# INFORMATION FOR ADOLESCENTS

*Candlelighters Teenage Newsletter* (Serial). Quarterly. Free

A quarterly newsletter written by and for adolescent cancer patients, containing personal narratives as well as information about programs and publications of interest to teenagers.

» *Teens Newsletter Candlelighters*
*National Headquarters*
*123 C St., S.E.*
*Washington, DC 20003*
*(202) 544-1696*

*Waiting for Johnny Miracle.* Alice Bach. 1980. $8.95.

A novel, written for adolescents about a 17-year-old girl with osteogenic sarcoma. It centers on her experiences and feelings and those of her twin sister, parents, other family members, and friends. The novel depicts the family's efforts to continue life as normally as possible, and on hospitalization, clinic visits, and the feelings of other teenage cancer patients.

» *Harper and Row Publishers, Inc.*
*10 East 53rd St.*
*New York, NY 10022*

*Too Old To Cry, Too Young to Die.* Edity Pendleton. 1980. $7.95

This book records the experiences of 35 teenagers and young adults who have had cancer. If offers nine case studies of cancer patients and quotes and tips from these and other teenage patients on such subjects as cancer treatment, dealing with hospitalization and treatment staff, reactions of family members, returning to school, hair loss, dating relapse, and death.

» *Thomas Nelson Publishers*
*P.O. Box 946*
*407 Seventh Ave., South*
*Nashville, TN 37203*

# INFORMATION FOR SIBLINGS

*When Your Brother or Sister Has Cancer.* L. A. Rudolph. 1980. Free

A brochure written for children from grade school age to early adolescence, designed to help the brothers and sisters of cancer patients deal with their feelings. Some of the most common feelings a sibling may experience, such as anger, worry, sadness, guilt, and jealousy are discussed in order to reassure the child that these are normal reactions to having a sick child in the family.

» *The Children's Orthopedic Hospital and Medical Center*
*Division of Pediatric Hematology/Oncology*
*4800 Sand Point Way, N.E.*
*P.O. Box C5371*
*Seattle, WA 98105*
*(206) 634-5427*

# INFORMATION FOR PARENTS

*Candlelighters National Newsletter.* Serial. Quarterly. Contact source

Information of interest to parents of childhood cancer patients is presented. Issues such as legislation to aid patients and their families, bibliographies, programs of national interest, overseas group activities, and general background on childhood cancer are included.

» *Candlelighters National Headquarters*
*123 C. St., S.E.*
*Washington, DC 20003*
*(202) 544-1696*

*Childhood Cancer: A Pamphlet for Parents.* S. E. Sallan; P. Newburger. 1978. Free (limited supply)

Facts about the diagnosis, treatment, and psychological aspects of childhood cancer are presented in a colorfully illustrated brochure for parents. Issues such as second opinions; drugs and their side effects; and what to tell the child, his siblings, and other people are covered.

» *Sidney Farber Cancer Institute*
*Cancer Control Program*
*44 Binney St.*
*Boston, MA 02115*
*(617) 732-3150*

*Children Die Too.* J. Johnson; S. M. Johnson. 1978. Contact source

The booklet briefly discusses emotions such as denial, guilt, anger, and depression which are commonly experienced by bereaved parents. Parents are advised on how to treat other family members and friends who were involved with the dead child.

» *Centering Corp.*
*Box 878*
*Council Bluffs, IA 51502*

*Children in Hospitals, Inc.* (Newsletter). Quarterly. M. K. Saphier, ed.

Support and advice are offered to parents of hospitalized children, with the goal of making the hospitalization as pleasant and nontraumatic as possible. The newsletter contains articles, reviews of books, pamphlets, movies, and media programs, members' letters, and announcements of society activities. Children in Hospitals publishes a listing of hospital policies regarding family contact in Boston area hospital.

» *Children in Hospitals, Inc.*
*31 Wilshire Park*
*Needham, MA 02192*

*Coping at Home with Cancer. For Parents, by a Parent.* N. Cottrell. 1977. $1

Advice is offered to other parents of childhood cancer patients by parents of a two-year-old boy who died of a brain tumor at home. Their personal account emphasizes ways in which parents can care for terminally ill children at home, giving both nursing care and emotional support. Practical hints are summarized, including management of visits to the hospital, preparation of oral medications, and organizing recreational activities.

» *The Children's Hospital, Inc.*
*ATT: CHA*
*345 N. Smith Ave.*
*St. Paul, MN 55102*
*(612) 298-8666*

*Coping with Prolonged Health Impairment in Your Child.* A. T. McCollum. 1975. $11.50
Based in part on experiences with patients and their families in the Yale Children's Clinical Research Center and the Yale Cystic Fibrosis Program, the book was prepared to help families enhance the quality of life for their child who is afflicted with a prolonged physical disorder. General guidelines for anticipating needs and planning solutions are discussed. The ways professionals can offer significant help to the child and family are described.

» *Little, Brown and Co.*
*200 West St.*
*Waltham, MA 02154*
*(617) 227-0730*

*Emotional Aspects of Childhood Cancer and Leukemia: A Handbook for Parents.* J. J. Spinetta; P. D. Spinetta; F. Kung; D. B. Schwartz. 1976. $.75
The emotions often experienced by parents whose children have cancer are discussed and the demands of illness upon a family are considered. The booklet describes in some detail the initial reaction to diagnosis, children's concepts of death, hospitalization, home care, and methods of communicating with the child.

» *Leukemia Society of America, Inc.*
*San Diego Chapter*
*326 Broadway, Mezzanine Suite*
*San Diego, CA 92101*
*(714) 239-7781*

*Home Care for Dying Children: A Manual for Parents.* D. G. Moldow; I. M. Martinson. 1979. $4
This book describes the concept of home care and explains the situations in which it is practical. Ideas about treatment, pain relief, the importance of enjoying life as much as possible, and the provisions necessary for home care are also discussed.

» *School of Nursing*
*Univ. of Minnesota*
*3313 Powell Hall*
*500 Essex St., SE*
*Minneapolis, MN 55455*
*(612) 376-1430*

*Nutrition for Children with Cancer*

*My Child Has An Ostomy.* The United Ostomy Association. Free.

» *The United Ostomy Association*
*2001 West Beverly Blvd.*
*Los Angeles, CA 90057*

*Living One Day At a Time (LODAT).* Oncology Handbook for Parents. B. Lederer. 1977. Free

This booklet is designed to help parents of children with cancer cope with the psychological and practical problems of the illness. Information is provided on common childhood cancers, and on various forms of treatment and responses. A table of commonly used drugs and their side effects is given. Advice is given on how to: relay medical instructions to the patient, handle relatives and friends, prepare for out- or in-patient visits to the hospital, and pay bills. Includes a glossary of relevant medical terms, a bibliography of materials for both parents and children, names of organizations that can help parents of children with cancer, and a brief profile of LODAT.

» *LODAT*
*P.O. Box 13154*
*Milwaukee, WI 53213*
*(414) 461-5347*

*Organization and Information Handbook for Parents Groups: 1977-1978.* Contact source

Parents are instructed on how to form self-help groups and develop other outreach activities. Methods for recruiting members, organizing meetings, developing promotional materials, and coordinating chapter efforts with the national movement are explained. Information on linking with the American Cancer Society and community resources is also provided.

» *Candlelighters National Headquarters*
*123 C St., S. E.*
*Washington, DC 20003*
*(202) 544-1696*

*Parents: When Your Preschooler is Hospitalized, Consider Yourself an Important Member of the Medical Team.* M. K. Saphier. Children in Hospitals, Inc. Newsletter: 1–8, Spring 1977; contact source

The emotional trauma of separation and its effects on the hospitalized preschooler's relationship with his family is analyzed. If parents are unable to stay with the child constantly, alternative strategies to alleviate the child's anxiety during periods of absence are given. Suggestions for incorporating the parents into the patient care team are given, and parents are advised of their rights in a hospital situation.

» *Children in Hospitals, Inc.*
*31 Wilshire Park*
*Needham, MA 02192*

*Pediatric Oncology Bibliography.* M. Sachs; P. Tharp, compilers. 1980. Free

Book, journal articles, and audio-visual materials are listed in this resource guide prepared for pediatric oncology patients, their families, and health care professionals. Divided by general subject areas, the bibliography includes a section on agencies and organizations that provide information on cancer.

» *At-Home Rehabilitation Program*
*University Hospitals Cancer Center*
*2074 Abington Rd.*
*Cleveland, OH 44106*
*(216) 444-3783*

*Radiation Therapy: A Family Handbook.* C. U. Marshall; P. Flumnerfelt. $2.50 plus postage and handling

This illustrated handbook attempts to answer those questions concerning treatment of the pediatric cancer patient that are most frequently asked by patients and their families. The first chapter briefly explains the function of each member of the oncology team, while subsequent chapters cover all aspects of radiation treatment including the development of a protocol, equipment used, and possible side effects of therapy.

» *Indiana University School of Medicine*
*Radiation Oncology Dept.*
*1100 West Michigan St.*
*Indianapolis, IN 46223*
*(317) 264-2524*

*Talking to Children About Death.* 1979. $1.50

Suggested guidelines for talking with children about death. Discusses various situations in which children may ask questions about death.

» *Superintendent of Documents*
*U.S. Government Printing Office*
*Washington, D.C. 20402*
*(202) 783-3238*
*Order No. DHEW (ADM) 79-838*

*Leukemia: A Guide to the Management of the Disease.* G. Taylor. Free

This brochure is an adaptation of a chapter from "Experiences with Childhood Cancer." It discusses both the emotional crises faced by the parents and siblings of a child with a life-threatening illness and the management of these crises by health care professionals. The roles and responsibilities of nurses, doctors, and others are outlined. Supportive agencies are listed.

» *Leukemia Society of America, Inc.*
*National Headquarters*
*800 Second Ave.*
*New York, NY 10017*
*(212) 573-8484*

*Leukemia and the Family.* 1977. $1.75

This brochure focuses on the emotional and social effects of childhood leukemia on both patient and family. Some practical and technical information directly related to the disease (such as home nursing care and drugs employed to treat leukemia) is presented, but the brochure is mainly devoted to such problems as social isolation, marital stress, emotional stress endured by the leukemic child, and various reactions to the diagnosis.

» *Association for the Study of Childhood Cancer*
*MCV Station*
*Box 762*
*Richmond, VA 23298*

*Acute Lymphoblastic Leukemia (ALL) of Childhood: A Pamphlet for Parents.* S. E. Sallan. 1975. Free

Directed to parents, the pamphlet presents basic information about acute lymphoblastic leukemia in children, its diagnosis and treatment, and the emotional implications for the child and the family. A glossary at the end explains technical terms.

» *Sidney Farber Cancer Institute*
*44 Binney St.*
*Boston, MA 02115*
*(617) 732-3000*

*When Your Child Goes to the Hospital.* 1977. Contact source

Television's Mister Rogers suggests ways for parents to help their children deal with their feelings about the hospital experience.

» *Family Communications*
*Let's Talk About It*
*4802 Fifth Ave.*
*Pittsburgh, PA 15213*
*(412) 687-2990*

*When Your Child Goes to the Hospital.* P. D. Pizzo. 1976. $.85

Designed to help parents cope with their child's hospitalization, the importance of psychologically preparing both themselves and the child. Recommended methods include choosing a doctor and a hospital; a pre-hospitalization visit with the child; and giving the child simple, honest answers to his questions. Suggested readings and questions to ask about the hospital are appended.

» *Superintendent of Documents*
*U.S. Government Printing Office*
*Washington, D.C. 20402*
*(202) 783-3238*
*Order No. DHEW 76-30092; GPO*
*017-091-00217-7*

*The Bereaved Parent.* H. S. Schiff. 1977. $1.98

Offers advice to parents who are facing the death of a child as well as those whose child has already died. Covers the day-to-day decisions like funeral arrangements, and the problems involved in rebuilding family relationships.

» *Crown Publishers, Inc.*
*One Park Ave.*
*New York, N.Y. 10016*
*(212) 532-9200*

*What You Need to Know. . . . 1979.* **Free**

Brochures containing information on the nature of cancer, sources of assistance, areas of research, and definitions of medical terms. One booklet covers cancer in a general fashion while six others address forms of cancer most commonly seen in children: Brain, Bone, Hodgkin's Disease, Non-Hodgkin's Lymphoma, Childhood Leukemia, and Wilm's Tumor.

» *National Cancer Institute*
  *Office of Cancer Communications*
  *Bldg. 31, Rm. 10A18*
  *9000 Rockville Pike*
  *Bethesda, MD 20205*

*Diet and Nutrition: A Resource for Parents of Children with Cancer.* Reprinted June 1981. **Free.**

Developed by the Diet, Nutrition and Cancer Program of the National Cancer Institute, this book is intended to serve as a source of information on the many aspects of diet and nutrition as it relates to children with cancer. It provides background information and suggestions for dealing with day to day problems. Contains information on special dietary modifications.

» *National Cancer Institute*
  *See address above*

*Young People with Cancer: A Handbook for Parents.* 1982. **Free**

An excellent book for parents providing information on cancer and how to cope with it. Gives tips for clinic visits and a drug chart listing possible side effects along with medical information and practical tips gathered from the experience of others.

» *National Cancer Institute*
  *See address above*

*Tending the Sick Child.* M. Sherman. 1977. **Free**

A realistic booklet written by the mother of a child with cancer. It deals with general nutrition and the specific problems of children with cancer. Includes easy recipes that appeal to children.

» *National Cancer Institute*
  *See address above*

# 6

## IMPROVING THE

## FOOD YOU EAT

You may realize that you need to make every bite count, but you may not know exactly how to pack extra calories and protein into the food you eat. Here are some how-to's for increasing the calorie and/or protein content of foods, recipes, and convenience products. They have worked for others, and they may work for you. Use them as a jumping-off point. Once you get the idea, you can begin to think up your own ways to increase the nutrient density of your favorite foods.

Try to make it an automatic response; every time you prepare food, think of something you can add to make it just a little more nutritious. If you make every bite a two-for-one proposition, you have to eat only half as much.

The section on spices and herbs will give you suggestions for making your meals more palatable. The skillful use of herbs and spices will increase the mealtime pleasure of your whole family and add a new taste dimension to even long-familiar recipes and menus (see Table 6-1, pp. 65-69.)

## Increasing calories

If you do not feel like eating much, try incorporating high-fat foods into your diet. Since fat contains nine calories per gram, you will get the greatest number of calories in the smallest amount of food.

*Whipped cream:* At approximately 75 calories per tablespoon,

whipped cream makes a decorative, high-calor
Use a dab of whipped cream on pudding, cust
tin, fruit, hot chocolate, cereal, hot or iced coff

*Sour cream:* A rounded tablespoon will add
your total intake. Use sour cream on meat, fru
rice, in dips, as a garnish in soups, and, o
potatoes.

*Butter or margarine:* A generous teaspoon of
will add an extra 45 calories to your diet. Spr
margarine on toast and bread, and add melted
etables, hot cereals, rice, pasta, or sliced meat.

*Mayonnaise:* At an even 100 calories per table
can have a calorie-amplifying effect on such foc
salads, sandwiches, sauces, and even as a garnish
vegetables, or molded salads.

*High carbohydrate foods:* Small servings of
foods also help supplement the number of calc
Keep high-carbohydrate snacks available so that
eating "just a little something," you can nibble o
sicles, cookies, granola, fruit-nut mixes, frozen d
high-calorie bread (see Recipe section) spread
amount of butter—all will help boost your cal
high-carbohydrate foods, such as sugar, honey,
molasses, and marshmallows can also be incorp
Croutons can be added to soups and salads. Alco
ories per gram (if you heat it, the calories burn off
of your favorite liquor on top of ice cream, fruit,

*Chopped nuts and bacon:* A strip of bacon contain
and 2 grams of protein; 2 tablespoons of choppe
to 100 calories, depending on the type of nuts. Nu
protein source. Try adding nuts or bacon to cas
toppings.

Don't attempt to eat large amounts of fat or car
sitting. Just adding a little extra off and on throug
make a significant difference in your total calorie

## Providing extra protein

If you have a poor appetite, or protein foods like n
to you, try increasing the protein content of you
nonbulky, high-protein foods like the following:

*Peanut butter:* One tablespoon of peanut butter provides 4 grams protein and 90 calories, so you get both a protein and calorie ost. Try serving peanut butter on sliced fruit, celery or carrot cks, or spread it on toast or crackers for a snack.

*Fortified milk:* One cup of milk contains approximately 9 grams of otein. Use milk instead of water to make soup, pudding, cocoa, cooked cereals. You can double the protein content of milk from to 18 grams by adding 5 tablespoons of dried skim milk powder an 8 ounce glass of milk. Chilling enhances the flavor. Use for-ied milk in any recipe that calls for milk or whenever possible.

*Dry milk powder:* One-fourth cup of dry milk powder will add 6 ams of protein to a recipe. Try adding a tablespoon or two to ked items, hot cereals, gravy, cream sauces, and casserole dishes.

*Cheese.* Every ounce of cheese contains approximately 7 grams of :otein. Adding $\frac{1}{2}$ cup of grated cheese to casseroles, sauces, eggs, ' vegetables can tack on an additional 14 grams of protein, and $\frac{1}{2}$ ip of creamed cottage cheese provides 15 grams with very little olume. Try melting cheese on toast for a quick high-protein snack. dd cheese or cottage cheese to pastina, rice, noodles, or potatoes.

*Eggs:* You can calculate another 7 grams of protein for every egg ou eat. Put extra eggs in cake, cookies, bread, pudding, eggnogs, nd sauces. Add finely chopped hard-boiled eggs to a salad, gravy, uce, vegetable, or casserole. A rich eggnog (see Recipe section) is r better for a coffee break than a soft drink or coffee.

*Meat, fish, or poultry:* An ounce of meat, fish, or poultry is equal ) 7 grams of protein. Adding a little extra meat to noodle or rice asseroles can contribute a significant amount of protein. Finely hopped meat can be a good protein source that you will not even otice in soup.

*Tofu.* A 2-inch square of tofu (soybean curd) will add 9 grams of igh quality protein to broth or salad. This bland Oriental specialty available in most supermarkets and can be used in many ways. ry dipping it in a batter and frying it in bite-sized pieces for a tasty nack.

*Yogurt:* A cup of fruit-flavored yogurt contains approximately 60 calories and 9 grams of protein. Have a cup of yogurt and a few rackers or cookies for a snack.

## Adding extra nutrition to convenience foods

ry adding some extra nutrition to convenience foods for a quick, asy-to-prepare meal or snack. Here are some examples:

*Prepare* Kraft's Deluxe Macaroni and Cheese according to the package directions, but stir in an extra $\frac{1}{4}$ cup of milk, 2 tablespoons of margarine, and $\frac{1}{2}$ cup of shredded cheese.

*When preparing* Stouffer's Escalloped Chicken and Noodle Casserole, sauté 1 cup of diced chicken in 2 tablespoons of margarine, and add it to the dish during the last 10 minutes of baking. Top the casserole with an extra $\frac{1}{2}$ cup of breadcrumbs mixed in 2 tablespoons of melted butter.

*Try adding* $\frac{1}{2}$ cup of grated cheddar cheese and 1 tablespoon of dry milk powder to corn muffin mix. Sprinkle the tops with wheat germ or finely chopped nuts before baking.

## HIGH-CALORIE, READY-MADE ITEMS

If you do not feel like cooking and have no one to prepare food for you, take a good look around a supermarket, delicatessen, bakery, or restaurant to see what ready-made dishes are available. Here are a few ideas:

Cheesecake
Danish pastries
Brownies
Health food mixes (dried fruits, nuts, and seeds)
Granola
Nuts
Peanut butter
Soft cheeses and cheese spreads
Chips and dips
Candy bars
Super-rich ice cream
Gatorade

Frozen entrees (Italian dishes, macaroni and cheese, meat with noodle dishes)
Ready-to-eat puddings, custards, or tapioca
Chunky soups
Frozen desserts
Pizza
Fast foods (Big Mac, Whopper, milkshakes)
Reuben sandwich
Monte Cristo sandwich
Grilled cheese sandwich

## High-calorie and high-protein snacks

The following is a list of some of the recipes contained in the Recipe Section of the book which can be made ahead and kept on hand or in the freezer for easy high-calorie or high-protein snacks. Remember, it is not necessary to eat a great volume of food daily to obtain sufficient calories and protein. What is important is selecting your food carefully, especially if you are not hungry or if you fill up rather quickly. Make sure that you make every bite count.

Cheese ball
Cheese spread
Spicy roasted pecans
Granola
Snack packs
Granola bars
Feta cheese triangles
Pizza pick-ups
Ever-ready muffins
High fiber bread
Cranberry-banana bread

Best banana bread
Pumpkin nut bread
Macaroni and cheese
Fruit sherbet
Velvety sherbet
Creamy lemon sherbet
Peanut butter cookies
Nut bars
Lemon pound cake
Bourbon pound cake

## Tips for freezing food

Prepare food in double portions, and freeze one for future use. This will save you time in the kitchen. Here are some suggestions to help you:

*Undercook* the portion you plan to freeze so it does not overcook when you reheat it.

*Cook the food quickly.* The less time food stands at temperatures between 45 degrees and 140 degrees the better. If food remains at these temperatures for more than 3 hours, it may not be safe to freeze. Hot food can be placed in the refrigerator if it does not raise the refrigerator temperature above 45 degrees. Freeze food as soon as it cools.

*Store food for the freezer in containers,* or wrap it in moisture and vapor-proof materials. When wrapping food for the freezer, press out the air, and wrap tightly. Then seal with tape.

*Label your food* and note the date you put it in the freezer. Plan to use frozen food within one month. The food will not spoil, but it does lose flavor.

*To prepare freezer dinners,* you can use foil trays from convenience foods or shape foil dividers to place in cake or pie pans. Fill the tray or pan with food, cover it tightly with foil, label, and freeze.

*Try the small foil casseroles* available in stores. They can go directly from freezer to oven.

*Freeze herbs and chopped onion* to add zest to sandwiches and casseroles. Wash the herbs and drain them. Then wrap them in foil or put them in a plastic bag. Put the package in a carton or glass jar, and store it in the freezer. Peel, wash, and quarter onions. Chop them, and scald for $1\frac{1}{2}$ minutes. Then chill in ice water. Drain the onions, wrap, and freeze.

## TABLE 6-1 DICTIONARY OF HERBS AND SPICES

Approximately ⅓ teaspoon ground herbs or 1 teaspoon dried herbs is equal in strength to 1 tablespoon fresh herbs.

| Herb or Spice | Form | Flavor | Uses |
|---|---|---|---|
| *Allspice* | Whole or ground | Blend of cinnamon, nutmeg, and cloves | Spices meat, fish, seafood dishes, soups, juices, fruits, spicy sauces, spinach, turnips, peas, red and yellow vegetables |
| *Anise* | Whole or ground | Aromatic, sweet licorice flavor | Sweet rolls, breads, fruit pies and fillings, sparingly in fruit, stews, shellfish dishes, carrots, beets, cottage cheese |
| *Basil, sweet* | Fresh, whole or ground | Aromatic, mild mint-licorice flavor | Meat, fish, seafood dishes, eggs, soups, stews, sauces, salads, tomato dishes, most vegetables, fruit compotes |
| *Bay* | Dried whole leaves, ground | Aromatic, woodsy, pleasantly bitter | Meat, game, poultry, stews, fish, shellfish, chowders, soups, pickled meats and vegetables, gravies, marinades |
| *Burnet* | Fresh, dried leaves | Delicate cucumber flavor | Soups, salads, dressings, most vegetables, beverages, as a garnish |
| *Caraway* | Whole or ground, seed | Leaves and root delicately flavored, seeds sharp and pungent | Beans, beets, cabbage soup, breads, cookies, dips, variety meats, casseroles, dressings, cottage cheese, cheese spreads, sauerbraten |
| *Cardamom* | Whole or ground, seed | Mild pleasant ginger flavor | Pastries, pies, cookies, jellies, fruit dishes, sweet potatoes, pumpkin |
| *Cayenne* | Ground | Blend of hottest chili peppers | Sparingly in sauces, meat or seafood dishes, casseroles, soups, curries, stews, Mexican recipes, vegetables, cottage and cream cheeses |

TABLE 6-1  DICTIONARY OF HERBS AND SPICES—Continued

Approximately $\frac{1}{3}$ teaspoon ground herbs or 1 teaspoon dried herbs is equal in strength to 1 tablespoon fresh herbs.

| Herb or Spice | Form | Flavor | Uses |
|---|---|---|---|
| Chervil | Fresh, whole | Delicate parsley flavor | Soups, salads, stews, meats, fish, garnishes, eggs, sauces, dressings, vegetables, cottage cheese |
| Chili powder | Powder | Blend of chillies and spices | Sparingly in Mexican dishes, meats, stews, soups, cocktail sauces, eggs, seafoods, relishes, dressings |
| Chives | Fresh, frozen, dried | Delicate onion flavor | As an ingredient or garnish for any dish complemented by this flavor |
| Cinnamon | Whole sticks or ground | Warm spicy flavor | Pastries, desserts, puddings, fruits, spiced beverages, pork, chicken, stews, sweet potatoes, carrots, squash |
| Cloves | Whole or ground | Hot, spicy, penetrating | Sparingly with pork, in soups, desserts, fruits, sauces, baked beans, candied sweet potatoes, carrots, squash |
| Coriander | Whole or ground, seed | Pleasant lemon-orange flavor | Pastries, cookies, cream or pea soups, Spanish dishes, dressings, spiced dishes, salads, cheeses, meats |
| Cumin | Ground, seed | Warm, distinctive, salty-sweet, reminiscent of caraway | Meat loaf, chili, fish, soft cheeses, deviled eggs, stews, beans, cabbage, fruit pies, rice, Oriental meat cookery |
| Curry | Powder | Combination of many spices, warm, fragrant, exotic, combinations vary | Meats, sauces, stews, soups, fruits, eggs, fish, shellfish, poultry, creamed and scalloped vegetables, dressings, cream or cottage cheeses |
| Dill | Fresh, dried (whole or ground), seed | Aromatic, somewhat like caraway, but milder and sweeter | Seafood, meat, poultry, spreads, dips, dressings, cream or cottage cheeses, potato salads, many vegetables, soups, chowders |

| | | | |
|---|---|---|---|
| *Fennel* | Fresh, dried (whole or ground), seed | Pleasant licorice flavor somewhat like anise | Breads, rolls, sweet pastries, cookies, apples, stews, pork, squash, eggs, fish, beets, cabbage |
| *Ginger* | Fresh whole root, ground, crystallized | Aromatic, sweet, spice, penetrating | Cakes, pies, cookies, chutneys, curries, beverages, fruits, meats, poultry, stews, yellow vegetables, beets, soups, dressings, cheese dishes |
| *Mace* | Whole or ground | This dried pulp of the nutmeg kernel has a strong nutmeg flavor | Chicken, creamed fish, fish sauces, cakes, cookies, spiced doughs, jellies, beverages, yellow vegetables, cheese dishes, desserts, toppings |
| *Marjoram* | Fresh, dried (whole or ground) | Faintly like sage, slight mint aftertaste, delicate | Pork, lamb, beef, game, fish, fish sauces, poultry, chowders, soups, stews, sauces, cottage or cream cheeses, omelets, soufflés, green salads, many vegetables |
| *Mint* | Fresh, dried | Fruity, aromatic, distinctive flavor | Lamb, veal, fish, soups, fruit, desserts, cottage or cream cheeses, sauces, salads, cabbage, carrots, beans, potatoes |
| *Mustard* | Fresh, dried (whole or ground) | Sharp, hot, very pungent | Salads, dressings, eggs, sauces, fish, spreads, soups, many vegetables |
| *Nutmeg* | Whole or ground | Spicy, sweet, pleasant | Desserts of all kinds, stews, sauces, cream dishes, soups, fruits, beverages, ground meats, many vegetables |
| *Oregano (wild marjoram)* | Fresh, dried (whole or ground) | More pungent than marjoram, but similar, reminiscent of thyme | Italian cooking, Mexican cooking, spaghetti, tomato sauces, soups, meats, fish, poultry, eggs, omelets, spreads, dips, many vegetables, green salads, mushroom dishes |

*Improving the Food You Eat*

## TABLE 6-1 DICTIONARY OF HERBS AND SPICES—Continued

Approximately $\frac{1}{4}$ teaspoon ground herbs or 1 teaspoon dried herbs is equal in strength to 1 tablespoon fresh herbs.

| Herb or Spice | Form | Flavor | Uses |
|---|---|---|---|
| Parsley | Fresh, dried flakes | Sweet, mildly spicy, refreshing | As a garnish, ingredient in soups, spreads, dips, stews, butters, all meats, poultry, fish, most vegetables, omelets, eggs, herb breads, salads |
| Poppy seed | Tiny, whole dried seed | Nut flavor | Breads, rolls, cakes, soups, cookies, dressings, cottage or cream cheeses, noodles, many vegetables, fruits, deviled eggs, stuffings |
| Rosemary | Fresh, whole | Refreshing, piny, resinous, pungent | Sparingly in meats, game, poultry, soups, fruits, stuffings, eggs, omelets, herb breads, sauces, green salads, marinades, vegetables |
| Saffron | Whole or ground | Exotic, delicate, pleasantly bittersweet | Expensive, but a little goes far; use for color and flavor in rice dishes, potatoes, rolls, breads, fish, stew, veal, chicken, bouillabaisse, curries, scrambled eggs, cream cheese, cream soups, sauces |
| Sage | Fresh, whole, or rubbed | Pungent, warm, astringent | Sparingly in pork dishes, fish, veal, lamb, stuffings, cheese dips, fish chowders, consommé, cream soups, gravies, green salads, tomatoes, carrots, lima beans, peas, onions, brussels sprouts, eggplant |
| Savory | Fresh, dried (whole or ground) | Warm, aromatic, resinous, delicate sage flavor, winter savory stronger than summer savory | Egg dishes, salads, soups, seafoods, pork, lamb, veal, poultry, tomatoes, beans, beets, cabbage, peas, lentils, summer squash, artichokes, rice, barbecue dishes, stuffings |
| Sesame | Whole seed | Toasted, it has a nutlike flavor | Breads, rolls, cookies, fish, lamb, eggs, fruit or vegetable salads, chicken, thick soups, vegetables, casseroles, toppings, noodles, candies |

*Nutrition and the Cancer Patient*

| | | | |
|---|---|---|---|
| *Tarragon* | Fresh, dried (whole or ground) | Licorice-anise flavor, pleasant, slightly bitter | Sparingly in egg dishes, fish, shellfish, veal, poultry, chowders, chicken, soups, butters, vinegar, sauces, marinades, beans, beets, cabbage, cauliflower, broccoli, vegetable juices, fresh sprigs in salads |
| *Thyme* | Fresh, dried (whole or ground) | Strong, pleasant, pungent clove flavor | Sparingly in fish, gumbo, shellfish, soups, meats, poultry, tomato juice or sauces, cheeses, eggs, sauces, fricasees, tomatoes, artichokes, beets, beans, mushrooms, potatoes, onions, carrots |
| *Tumeric* | Whole or ground | Aromatic, warm, mild | Substitutes for saffron in salads, salad dressings, butters, creamed eggs, fish, curries, rich dishes without saffron, vegetables, used partially for its orange color |
| *Watercress* | Fresh | Pleasing, peppery | Garnish or ingredient in salads, fruit or vegetable cocktails, soups, cottage cheese, spreads, egg dishes or sprinkled on vegetables or salads |

# Using herbs and spices

The skillful use of herbs and spices will increase the mealtime pleasure of your whole family and add a new taste dimension to even long-familiar recipes and menus.

Unsalted foods are more tasty if they are flavored with herbs and spices, which you can learn to use as easily as salt and pepper.

Table 6-1 suggests which combinations of herbs go best with particular foods. In cooking with herbs, remember that they should accentuate, not overpower, the flavor of your food. Use them discreetly. If you follow the rules listed below, you should be successful. It is a good rule of thumb to plan just one strongly seasoned dish per meal.

1. Use no more than $\frac{1}{4}$ teaspoon of dried herbs or $\frac{3}{4}$ teaspoon of fresh herbs for a dish that serves four. Start with that amount, then increase it to suit your taste.
2. Add herbs during the last hour of cooking to soups and stews that must be cooked a long time.
3. Add herbs before cooking hamburgers, meat loaf, and stuffing.
4. Sprinkle herbs on roasts before cooking, or top with herb-flavored margarine after cooking.
5. Steaks and chops can either be sprinkled with herbs while the meat is cooking or brushed with oil and sprinkled with herbs one hour before cooking.
6. Add herbs to vegetables, sauces, or gravies while they are cooking. If you wish, moisten the herbs first with a small amount of oil and let them stand half an hour, before adding them.
7. Add herbs several hours before serving cold foods, such as tomato juice, salad dressing, and cottage cheese. These foods can be stored in the refrigerator for three or four hours or overnight to enhance their flavor.
8. To bring out the essence of the herbs in your food, put the dried herbs in a tea strainer and dip the strainer into piping hot water for 20 seconds. After draining, add the moistened herbs to your food. (Heat and moisture bring out the fragrance and flavor of dried herbs.)
9. If you do not want bits of herbs in the food, tie the herbs in a small piece of cheesecloth and remove the bag before serving.
10. Combine herbs with margarine to flavor steaks, roasts, or vegetables after cooking.
11. If your diet allows it, marinate meats in a wine and herb mixture before cooking.
12. Crush dried herbs in the palm of your hand before adding them to your food. This hastens the flavor release.

13. When substituting fresh herbs for dried herbs, use three or four times the amount specified.
14. Do not combine too many herbs and spices in one dish, even though many would complement it.

The correct combination of herbs and spices for any food is the one that tastes best to you. Remember that seasoning foods is not a science but an expressive art—and you are the artist. When experimenting with a new herb, crush some of it and let it warm in your hand; then sniff it and taste it. If it is delicate, you can be bold and adventurous. If it is very strong and pungent, be cautious.

# 7

## SOME SPECIAL

## SITUATIONS

## YOU MAY FACE

Many types of cancer are now considered chronic illnesses, not acute fatal diseases. Long-term management and treatment may present you with a wide spectrum of problems and situations that must be recognized, addressed, and dealt with. You need to consider all the ramifications of your illness: financial problems, the psychological impact on your family and friends, and the effect on your work situation, as well as your treatment and nutritional status. You may feel that you would like to be left alone, or bury your head in the sand, or disappear for a while—a quite normal reaction in which you are not alone. Take strength from the support groups available to you, and plan workable solutions so you can achieve a satisfying quality of life.

The directions and goals you had prior to your diagnosis may shift dramatically. Many priorities are going to change, and old values may be altered. This is to be expected. Just don't flounder or drift. You will be happier and more successful if you give some thought to your new goals, based on your new needs, and work in a realistic framework so that you and those you love will not be at odds.

### "I just can't cope"

Not in the least unusual. There are many people who find it hard to cope with far less serious situations. When you feel you are not coping well, don't hesitate to seek professional help. For example, when you find it difficult to control your emotional responses, when your treatment is so difficult you want to quit, when you can't find anyone who understands or is willing to talk about your problems—seeking professional help can make a world of difference for you and your loved ones. Reaching out for help does not come naturally to us in this modern world, which tends to emphasize "pulling yourself up by your bootstraps" and prizes single-handed accomplishments. So you will have to make a conscious effort to obtain the help you need, just as you must consciously maintain your nutritional status.

There are many groups and agencies dedicated to helping people like you, and they can make this difficult time in your life much easier. Chapter 9 contains a listing of some of them, and your medical team or your local American Cancer Society will also be able to suggest a therapist or local self-help group.

## Well-meaning family and friends

Most of us have concerned family and friends who care and want to contribute whatever they can to make life easier for us, particularly when we are ill. However, depression, anxiety, or self-consciousness, coupled with cultural norms that encourage self-sufficiency, may lead us to withdraw and reject offers of help in times of trouble.

This can be particularly difficult when concerned family and friends pressure you to eat. Try to remember that it is love that motivates them. Explain that you appreciate their concern, but constant coaxing and cajoling only make matters worse. It is very difficult for someone with a normal appetite to understand why you do not feel like eating—especially when they know it is so important. Their continual urging is the result of the frustration they feel at standing by, unable to do anything.

It is heartbreaking to sit on the sidelines feeling there is nothing you can do to help someone you care about when that person is in obvious need. Before long, the natural response will be to avoid the frustrating situation. Don't feel you are imposing on your family and friends by letting them help. They want to. They just need a little guidance from you.

Try a constructive way to get out from under these pressures: find ways to let others help you. They will feel better if you suggest some supportive tasks they can do to help you. Let them do your shopping, run tiring errands, or take you to your appointment with the doctor. Allow them to purchase or prepare food to have on hand when you do feel like eating. If you are the family cook, let friends help you by cooking for your family on treatment days or when you are not feeling well. All of you will be more comfortable when you are together if your family and friends can make a definite, visible contribution which is of real value to you.

## The discomfort of those around you

Another situation you may have to face is others' inability to deal with your condition. You may find that when you return to work or school, people are uneasy or awkward about approaching you. Some people are threatened by discussion of any illness. You need to be sensitive to this and recognize this reaction for what it is—a personal fear and denial—not a purposeful avoidance or rejection of you.

Others may not be sure what to say or how to say it and may avoid mentioning your disease rather than say anything to upset or embarrass you. The best thing to do is to set the tone yourself— whether you want to talk about your illness, ignore the issue completely, or discuss only certain aspects. Let people know right away what you do or do not want to discuss and whether you are sensitive about certain things. Share your concerns and insecurities with those closest to you. Your family and friends have your best interests at heart, but they need direction on the best way to relate to you.

Because your life and your outlook on it have changed dramatically, you may have to learn very quickly to relate in a totally new way. It is not unusual to feel that your relationships are all slightly skewed: no statement comes out right, all actions are misinterpreted. If everyone—including you—seems edgy or overly sensitive or insensitive, you may consider retreating completely. This is the time to initiate your personal outreach program. Call your local American Cancer Society for the name of a self-help group near you or seek professional counseling.

## No time to eat on treatment days

Logistical problems can be an obstacle to meeting your basic nutrition needs. If you are receiving treatment several times a week, you may find you are consistently missing meals, particularly if you do not want to eat before treatment and end up waiting several hours for treatment to start. By the time you are finished, you may be exhausted and harried at best, even if you do not incur side effects. When you get home in the evening, you may be unable to eat. Under the rigors of this schedule, malnutrition is a real possibility.

You can prevent this downward spiral by planning ahead. Work out a system that is convenient, practical, and realistic for you.

### Suggestions

*Get up a little earlier* to leave time for eating or drinking a bland meal before you set out.

*Take a nutritious snack with you,* one that is light, easily carried, and convenient to eat, wherever you happen to be waiting. Some snacks that might fill the bill are peanut butter and crackers, cheese and crackers, a bag of nuts, a hearty soup in a thermos, a peanut butter and jelly sandwich, a can of complete nutritional supplement, or a package of Instant Breakfast that can be added to a carton of milk.

*Don't just sit around in the waiting room.* Ask how long the wait for treatment will be, and find a park, cafeteria, or luncheonette where you can go and relax with a nutritious snack.

## When you have to prepare food for your family

All too often, wives and mothers feel an obligation to keep things going as before. You may have to break old habit patterns for a while if you are the family cook—particularly if you enjoy cooking and pride yourself on it. There may be times when you will not feel like chopping, dicing, or sautéing onions, garlic, or peppers, or preparing savory stews redolent with herbs. Streamline your routines when you are tired or queasy, and learn to share or delegate the work. You may discover some new tricks that will serve you well in the future.

### Suggestions

*Always vent the cooking area with an exhaust fan.*

*Prepare foods with minimum aroma.*

*Make several dishes at once,* and cook them in the oven while you lie down and rest in a room away from kitchen odors.

*Freeze individual portions of food* to have on hand when you don't feel like cooking.

*Make double or triple batches of recipes when you feel good,* and store or freeze them. (See Chapter 6 for freezing instructions.)

*Make use of utensils that smother odors and save labor.* A microwave oven, a crock pot, a clay pot, or cooking in foil can be invaluable tools for the cook who is not feeling well.

*Let your family and friends help you.* When people extend offers of help, let them cook for your family on your treatment days or prepare a meal you can put in your freezer. Even small children can have a genuine growth experience if you just let them show what they can do.

*Use convenience and packaged foods* that are easy to prepare.

*Eat out occasionally* or get "take-out" foods for days when you are especially tired.

*If you feel best in the morning,* do all the preparation for the evening meal then, so you can pop it in the oven at dinnertime. The recipes for Summer Garden Chicken, Beef and Beer Casserole, and Macaroni and Cheese lend themselves to this schedule (see Recipe Index).

## Facing an unwanted meal

Trying to eat when you simply are not hungry or feel queasy and nauseous can be a formidable trauma. Some of the suggestions outlined here may help you overcome your reluctance to eat.

### Suggestions

*Make an effort to relax before meals.* Find ways to make yourself more receptive to eating. Relaxation techniques can help. If it is not contraindicated (ask your doctor) a pre-meal glass of sherry or wine may help ease tension and/or pain and stimulate appetite. Alternatively you may want to ask your physician for a mild tranquilizer or relaxant.

*Freshen up* before sitting down to eat. Wash your face, and use a mouthwash to get rid of any sour taste in your mouth which might distort the taste of food. Changing clothes may put you in a more upbeat frame of mind.

*Eat in your favorite room*—never in the food preparation area.

*Use nice plates and attractive serving dishes*—never containers, cans, or cartons used for storage or preparation of food.

*If distraction helps,* watch television, converse with others, or read a book while you are eating.

*Don't be overly worried* about marginal intake. Do the best you can on bad days, and make up for nutritional losses on better days.

*Focus on meeting your protein and calorie needs.* This is not the time to worry about cholesterol or a specific number of servings from the basic four food groups.

*On days when you are very ill,* your primary goal should be to meet your fluid requirements and avoid dehydration and electrolyte problems.

*If eating triggers nausea, vomiting, or diarrhea,* you must handle the problem days pragmatically, in the best way you can. Some prefer not to eat at all when they are symptomatic. Others eat bland, innocuous food that will not be any worse coming up than it was going down.

# 8

## ALTERNATIVE THERAPIES

Purveyors of worthless health cures have been around for a long time and will doubtless be with us forever. All too often, cancer patients and their families are the targets of unscrupulous charlatans who play on fear, lack of information, and, regrettably, real or imagined insensitivity of health professionals to their patients' needs. In a vain attempt to find comfort, hope, or an alternative to unpleasant treatments, many spend countless dollars and valuable treatment time on unproven therapies which often feature a nutritional component. If you are tempted to take a chance with a questionable method or practitioner, remember that over a million and a half living Americans have been cured of cancer by early diagnosis and prompt treatment with proven methods of surgery, radiation, and chemotherapy.

In the history of medicine, important advances have often been developed from obscure beginnings, and cancer researchers eagerly follow every lead that suggests a cure, no matter where it originates. However, the medical profession rightly insists on reliable standards for proof of efficacy and safety for any treatments proposed in the treatment of human beings. The scientific community

NOTE: The information in this chapter is based on material published by the American Cancer Society and on an article entitled "Unproved Dietary Claims In the Treatment of Patients with Cancer," written by M. E. Shils, M.D., and M. G. Hermann, R.D., published in the *Bulletin of the New York Academy of Medicine*, 2d series, vol. 58, no. 3, pp. 323–340, April 19, 1982.

cannot possibly investigate every suggestion, no matter how well-meaning, that is offered to the lay public. Generally accepted, standard research techniques are used as guidelines, and open communication and cooperation are actively practiced by those truly interested in curing and treating cancer.

The National Cancer Institute and the American Cancer Society are anxious to help you. If you have a question about a method that has been proposed to you, call the Cancer Information Service or your local American Cancer Society to see if they have any information on it. See Chapter 8 for telephone numbers.

## Hallmarks of the charlatan

Literally thousands of worthless cancer "remedies," embracing a wide range of materials, methodologies, and rationales, have been promoted and sold in the nineteenth and twentieth centuries alone. Slick advertising promotes these "cures" in unscientific books, magazines, and advertisements. Had any worked better than the established regimes, we would not have a new crop of remedies appearing each year.

Because it is often difficult to recognize purveyors of unorthodox "cures," the American Cancer Society has made a list of characteristics that distinguish those who promote unproven methods of cancer management:

1. They tend to be isolated from established scientific facilities or associates.
2. They do not use regular channels of communication (current, reputable medical journals) for reporting scientific information.
3. They claim organized medicine hinders their efforts because it is prejudiced against them.
4. They are prone to attack prominent scientists with bitter criticism.
5. They are quick to cite examples of physicians and scientists in the past who fought a noble fight against the rigid dogma of their day.
6. They strengthen their case by using complex jargon and unusual phraseology.
7. Their records are scanty or nonexistent.
8. They discourage or even refuse consultation with reputable physicians; and if their methods are scientifically evaluated, they generally decline to accept the results, claiming that the "medical trust" is against them.

9. The method of treatment is available only from them, and it is often secret. Alternately, the mode of administration depends on special judgment which can be learned only from them.
10. They discount biopsy verification in cancer diagnosis, sometimes by saying that it "spreads" the cancer (untrue). They may accept patients who have already been cured of cancer by orthodox means, but who fear they are not cured.
11. They may use proven drugs or other methods of treatment as adjuncts to the unproven therapy. If a favorable effect on cancer is shown, they will claim that it is a result of their unproven method.
12. They may display multiple and unusual degrees, such as N.D. (Doctor of Naturopathy), Ph.N. (Philosopher of Naturopathy), Ms.D. (Doctor of Metaphysics). These degrees have often been awarded by correspondence schools. For their testimonials, they feature people who are not trained or experienced in the natural history of cancer, the care of patients, or scientific methodology, such as actors, writers, statesmen, lawyers, or other prominent citizens or celebrities outside the medical profession.

Who, you might ask, would want to entrust his or her life to the promoter of an unproven method? Primarily those who hold the erroneous belief that all cancer is incurable, and who consequently cannot see the logic of undergoing conventional treatments which may have side effects. This group seems to feel that since nothing works, they have nothing to lose and that miracle cures, or "natural treatments," which are often billed as "painless," are preferable to the proven methods. This attitude is especially self-defeating today, when more and more cancers are treated successfully, and when ongoing long-term management has restored two out of five people with cancer to a normal life five years after the diagnosis of their disease.

Some people fear the financial burden of cancer; and since many fraudulent cure therapies do not require hospitalization or repeated visits to a hospital or clinic, they look financially desirable. The fact is that the unproven treatments may be more costly, not only financially, but also medically, because the disease process continues to advance while unsuccessful treatments are tried. Often the disease has progressed too far to be effectively treated ·by conventional means when professional help is finally sought.

Grasping at straws is a normal human reaction in a seemingly helpless, overwhelming situation, and unfortunately there are many exploiters who take advantage of this attitude. As long as there are frightened buyers, there will be charming, emotionally supportive miracle workers to take their money and promise anything they want to hear.

## Mythical nutrition "cures"

Recent miracle claims based on nutrition include megavitamin therapy, diet manipulation, "genating" the cells, correcting "metabolic imbalances," "detoxification," and the use of so-called antitumor agents, such as laetrile (so-called $B_{17}$) and pangamic acid (so-called $B_{15}$).

### LAETRILE

When laetrile was investigated by several leading medical centers, including Memorial Sloan-Kettering Cancer Center, the Mayo Clinic, the University of Arizona, and UCLA, it was found to be totally ineffective in checking abnormal cell growth. In fact, depending on the dose, it has been found that cyanide released from orally ingested laetrile may be toxic.

### DETOXIFICATION

Promoters of detoxification claim that "toxins" caused by the tumor make you feel sick and that "flushing them out" requires periodic fasting, purges, and colonic enemas. No reputable clinician has ever detected tumor toxins which cause such adverse reactions. Even if such toxins were present, they could be handled by the efficient function of the liver and kidneys, which process high-volume loads resulting from normal metabolism and destruction of cancer cells. The alternate flushing and starving methods used in detoxification can deplete valuable nutrients and weaken the body further.

### PANCREATIC ENZYMES

Another popular practice involves the use of pancreatic enzymes to "digest" the cancerous cells and to "restore" the level of pancreatic enzymes which proponents of this method claim are lowered in cancer. There are several fallacies in this basic premise. First, cancer is not associated with lower levels of pancreatic secretions except in cancer of the pancreas. Second, pancreatic enzymes are not designed to be activated in any part of the body except in the upper intestinal tract, where their job is to break down food products. Consequently, ingested enzymes will be hydrolyzed and inactivated in the upper intestinal tract and will never reach the site of the tumor. They are ineffective, since they cannot be absorbed in the bloodstream, and are potentially dangerous, since they are capable of eroding tissue that should not be exposed to them.

## MEGAVITAMINS

Vitamins are necessary for basic metabolic activities, but only in small or minute amounts. Once a particular vitamin requirement is met, the body either stores the excess or excretes it in the urine. Fat-soluble vitamins—A, D, E, and K—are stored in the body, and excessive amounts may create toxicity or other adverse effects. Sometimes excess vitamins actually inhibit or work against particular chemotherapeutic agents. No vitamin preparation should be taken without the consent of your physician or oncologist.

# How to protect yourself

If you are unhappy with your treatment or your physician, don't hesitate to go to another doctor. If you are unsure where to go, call the Cancer Information Service (800) 638-6694 or your local American Cancer Society chapter to find an oncologist or treatment center near you.

Feel free to ask your physician any question, to discuss any problem you might have, or to ask for a second opinion at any time during your treatment. If the physician you are seeing does not fulfill your needs, don't be embarrassed to change doctors. Be sure to inform the doctor so your records can be forwarded to the new doctor. This will avoid the expense of repeating tests and X-rays. However, if several qualified physicians give you the same opinion, don't try to second-guess your situation by continuing to go from one doctor to another. Select a doctor and a treatment program that you are comfortable with, and cooperate with your medical team. Above all, do not let yourself be fooled into believing in a painless, quick cure by a quack whose lucrative business is derived from desperate patients and families. Check out any doctor or treatment with your county medical society or local American Cancer Society.

Be leery of anyone (1) who promises a sure cure, when others do not; (2) whose treatment is secret, available only to himself; (3) whose treatment is advertised, usually under his own name or under a high-sounding label; (4) who claims to be persecuted by the medical profession; (5) whose chief supporters are nonmedical people; (6) who declines to consult with reputable physicians.

There are cures, and there are miracles. But you will not find them by submitting yourself to an unproven method of therapy promoted by a charlatan.

# 9

## OUTREACH: SOURCES OF
## HELP AND INFORMATION

When you are faced with a grave medical problem, you must be as aggressive in your approach to emotional and intellectual support as you are in your nutrition program. You need to make a deliberate effort to reach out and find the support groups which will be of maximum benefit to you—and there are many to choose from.

Start by asking your oncologist and the other members of your medical team any and all the questions you have, even if you feel they are not strictly medical. As professionals with an ongoing, daily involvement with the disease, they have doubtless confronted most of the issues that concern you many times before. Furthermore, most medical professionals are committed to treat the whole person. If they cannot come up with an answer, they will probably be able to steer you to the appropriate agency or support group.

The National Cancer Institutes, Office of Cancer Communications (301) 496-5583 or 496-6631, is an excellent hotline for information and referral, as is your local chapter of the American Cancer Society. Both can also send you lists of their publications. The publications listed on the following pages of this book deal primarily with nutrition, but there are many others available, covering all aspects of cancer.

### Comprehensive cancer centers

Either you or your doctor can call the nearest Comprehensive Cancer Center or the National Cancer Institutes with questions about your treatment or to find out what the newest/best treatment is and whether it is generally available. It is probably not necessary to consult them for the most common types of cancer, as you can receive excellent treatment in your home community if your physician is aware of the latest methods. However, if you want a second opinion, or if the physician or hospital where you will be treated sees relatively few cases of the type of cancer you have, you may want to call to verify the type of treatment prescribed.

Most Comprehensive Cancer Centers utilize the most up-to-date treatment programs available and are also involved in research studies to test the most promising new methods. In these studies, the control group receives the treatment currently considered best for the particular type of cancer, and the test group receives an experimental treatment that may turn out to be even more effective. Because these studies are federally financed clinical trials, your medical expenses may be partly or completely covered if you participate. The toll-free Cancer Information Service can put you in touch with the trials in your area (800) 638-6694.

ALABAMA
Comprehensive Cancer Center
University of Alabama in
　Birmingham
University Station
Birmingham, AL 35294
(205) 934-5077

CALIFORNIA
Los Angeles County—University
　of Southern California Compre-
　hensive Cancer Center
2025 Zonal Avenue
Los Angeles, CA 90033
(213) 226-2008

UCLA Cancer Center
UCLA School of Medicine
924 Westwood Boulevard, Suite 650
Los Angeles, CA 90024
(213) 825-1532
(213) 825-5268

CONNECTICUT
Yale University Comprehensive
　Cancer Center
333 Cedar Street
New Haven, CT 06510
(203) 432-4122

DISTRICT OF COLUMBIA
Georgetown University/Howard
　University
Comprehensive Cancer Center
Vincent T. Lombardi Cancer
　Research Center
Georgetown University Medical
　Center
3800 Reservoir Road, N.W.
Washington, DC 20007
(202) 625-7066

Howard University Cancer
　Research Center
College of Medicine
Washington, DC 20059
(202) 745-1406

FLORIDA
Comprehensive Cancer Center for
　the State of Florida
University of Miami School of
　Medicine/Jackson Memorial
　Medical School
P.O. Box 016960
Miami, FL 33101
(305) 547-6758

ILLINOIS
Illinois Cancer Council
36 S. Wabash Avenue, Suite 700
Chicago, IL 60603
(312) 346-9813

MARYLAND
Johns Hopkins Oncology Center
601 North Broadway
Baltimore, MD 21205
(301) 955-8822

MASSACHUSETTS
Sidney Farber Cancer Institute
44 Binney Street
Boston, MA 02115
(617) 732-3555

MICHIGAN
Comprehensive Cancer Center of
  Metropolitan Detroit
110 East Warren Avenue
Detroit, MI 48201
(313) 833-0710

MINNESOTA
Mayo Comprehensive Cancer
  Center
200 First Street, S.W.
Rochester, MN 55901
(507) 284-2511

NEW YORK
Cancer Center/Institute of Cancer
  Research
Columbia University
701 W. 168th Street
New York, NY 10032
(212) 694-3807

Memorial Sloan-Kettering Cancer
  Center
1275 York Avenue
New York, NY 10021
(212) 794-7585

Roswell Park Memorial Institute
666 Elm Street
Buffalo, NY 14263
(716) 845-5770

NORTH CAROLINA
Comprehensive Cancer Center
Duke University Medical Center
P.O. Box 3814
Durham, NC 27710
(919) 684-2282

OHIO
Ohio State University Comprehensive Cancer Center
357 McCampbell Drive
Columbus, OH 43201
(614) 422-5022

PENNSYLVANIA
Fox Chase/University of
  Pennsylvania
Comprehensive Cancer Center
The Fox Chase Cancer Center
7701 Burholme Avenue
Philadelphia, PA 19111
(215) 342-1000

University of Pennsylvania Cancer
  Center
578 Maloney Building
3400 Spruce Street
Philadelphia, PA 19104
(215) 662-3910

TEXAS
The University of Texas System
  Cancer Center
M.D. Anderson Hospital and
  Tumor Institute
6723 Bertner Drive
Houston, TX 77030
(713) 792-3000

WASHINGTON
Fred Hutchinson Cancer Research
  Center
1124 Columbia Street
Seattle, WA 98104
(206) 292-2930

WISCONSIN
The University of Wisconsin Clinical Cancer Center
1300 University Avenue
Madison, WI 53706
(608) 263-2553

# Cancer Information Services

Cancer Information Services (CIS) offices are affiliated with Comprehensive Cancer Centers (special research and treatment centers recognized by the National Cancer Institute) and with the American Cancer Society.

CIS offices do not diagnose cancer or recommend treatment for individual cases. They do provide support, understanding, and rapid access to the latest information on cancer and local resources.

Telephone information may be supplemented by printed materials. All calls are kept confidential and you do not need to give your name.

For answers to questions about cancer, call the number for your state listed below.

Alaska: 800-638-6070
California: 800-252-9066 (from area codes 213, 714, and 805 only)
Connecticut: 800-922-0824
Delaware: 800-523-3586
District of Columbia: 636-5700
Florida: 800-432-5953
Georgia: 800-327-7332
Hawaii, Oahu: 524-1234
Hawaii, Neighbor Islands: Ask operator for Enterprise 6702
Illinois: 800-972-0586
Kentucky: 800-432-9321
Maine: 800-225-7034
Maryland: 800-492-1444
Massachusetts: 800-952-7420
Minnesota: 800-582-5262
New Hampshire: 800-225-7034
New Jersey, Northern: 800-223-1000
New Jersey, Southern: 800-523-3586
New York State: 800-462-7255
New York City: (212) 794-7982
North Carolina: 800-672-0943
North Dakota: 800-328-5188
Ohio: 800-282-6522
Pennsylvania: 800-822-3963
South Dakota: 800-328-5188
Texas: 800-392-2040
Vermont: 800-225-7034
Washington: 800-552-7212
Wisconsin: 800-362-8038
For all other states: 800-638-6694

# American Cancer Society

The American Cancer Society provides numerous national and local services, including three national services and rehabilitation programs. These programs are designed to help you learn more about your disease and its treatment and to provide psychological and social support. I Can Cope, CanSurmount, and the Cancer Adjustment Program are open to everyone. Information on them is available from your state chapter of the American Cancer Society. The I Can Cope program is a patient/family education program available in large clinics and hospitals. CanSurmount is a program run by cancer patients who are trained to help other cancer patients adjust to the physical, psychological, and social problems brought on by their condition. The Cancer Adjustment Program is a flexible service of group counseling and individual crisis intervention which focuses primarily on emotional and social problems.

In 1980, more than 400,000 people with cancer participated in the various American Cancer Society rehabilitation programs. Over 80,000 people were helped in the adjustment to laryngectomy, mastectomy, and ostomy rehabilitation.

Local American Cancer Society units are involved in basic service programs which include: (1) information and guidance for the patient and the family on how to make the best use of the American Cancer Society services, community health services, and other resources; (2) loans of sick-room supplies (e.g., hospital beds and wheelchairs) and special comfort items for the homebound patient; (3) surgical dressings prepared by volunteers; (4) transportation to and from a doctor's office, clinic, or hospital for treatment; (5) information on financial problems; (6) information on physician referrals; (7) booklets and pamphlets written about specific types of cancer, treatment, rehabilitation, and so on.

Depending on local policies and resources, American Cancer Society programs may include more expensive services, such as home care programs, blood programs, and childhood cancer programs.

The national headquarters provides assistance to all cancer patients and can help refer you to its specific programs: American Cancer Society, Inc., 777 Third Avenue, New York, NY 10017.

## CHARTERED DIVISIONS OF THE AMERICAN CANCER SOCIETY, INC.

ALABAMA DIVISION INC.
2926 Central Avenue
Birmingham, AL 35209
(205) 879-2242

ALASKA DIVISION, INC.
1343 G Street
Anchorage, AK 99501
(907) 277-8696

ARIZONA DIVISION, INC.
634 West Indian School Road
P.O. Box 33187

Phoenix, AZ 85067
(602) 264-5861

ARKANSAS DIVISION, INC.
5520 West Markham Street
P.O. Box 3822
Little Rock, AR 72203
(501) 664-3480,1,2

CALIFORNIA DIVISION, INC.
1710 Webster Street
Oakland, CA 94612
(415) 893-7900

COLORADO DIVISION, INC.
1809 East 18th Avenue
P.O. Box 18268
Denver, CO 80218
(303) 321-2464

CONNECTICUT DIVISION, INC.
Barnes Park South
14 Village Lane
P.O. Box 410
Wallingford, CT 06492
(203) 265-7161

DELAWARE DIVISION, INC.
Academy of Medicine Building
1925 Lovering Avenue
Wilmington, DE 19806
(302) 654-6267

DISTRICT OF COLUMBIA DIVI-
SION, INC.
Universal Building, South
1825 Connecticut Avenue, N.W.
Washington, D.C. 20009
(202) 483-2600

FLORIDA DIVISION, INC.
1001 South MacDill Avenue
Tampa, FL 33609
(813) 253-0541

GEORGIA DIVISION, INC.
1422 Peachtree Street, N.W.
Atlanta, GA 30309
(404) 892-0026

HAWAII DIVISION, INC.
Community Services Center
Building
200 North Vineyard Boulevard
Honolulu, HI 96817
(808) 531-1662,3,4,5

IDAHO DIVISION, INC.
1609 Abbs Street
P.O. Box 5386
Boise, ID 83705
(208) 343-4609

ILLINOIS DIVISION, INC.
37 South Wabash Avenue
Chicago, IL 60603
(312) 372-0472

INDIANA DIVISION, INC.
4755 Kingsway Drive, Suite 100
Indianapolis, IN 46205
(317) 257-5326

IOWA DIVISION, INC.
Highway #18 West
P.O. Box 980
Mason City, IO 50401
(515) 423-0712

KANSAS DIVISION, INC.
3003 Van Buren Street
Topeka, KS 66611
(913) 267-0131

KENTUCKY DIVISION, INC
Medical Arts Building
1169 Eastern Parkway
Louisville, KY 40217
(502) 459-1867

LOUISIANA DIVISION, INC.
Masonic Temple Building, Room
810
333 St. Charles Avenue
New Orleans, LA 70130
(504) 523-2029

MAINE DIVISION, INC.
Federal and Green Streets
Brunswick, ME 04011
(207) 729-3339

MARYLAND DIVISION, INC.
200 East Joppa Road
Towson, MD 21204
(301) 828-8890

MASSACHUSETTS DIVISION,
INC.
247 Commonwealth Avenue
Boston, MA 02116
(617) 267-2650

MICHIGAN DIVISION, INC.
1205 East Saginaw Street
Lansing, MI 48906
(517) 371-2920

MINNESOTA DIVISION, INC.
2750 Park Avenue
Minneapolis, MN 55407
(612) 871-2111

MISSISSIPPI DIVISION, INC.
345 North Mart Plaza
Jackson, MS 39206
(601) 362-8874

MISSOURI DIVISION, INC.
715 Jefferson Street
P.O. Box 1066
Jefferson City, MO 65101
(314) 636-3195

MONTANA DIVISION, INC.
2820 First Avenue South
Billings, MT 59101
(406) 252-7111

NEBRASKA DIVISION, INC.
Overland Wolfe Centre
6910 Pacific Street, Suite 210
Omaha, NE 68106
(402) 551-2422

NEVADA DIVISION, INC.
4100 Boulder Highway
Suite A
Las Vegas, NV 89121
(702) 454-4242

NEW HAMPSHIRE DIVISION,
INC.
686 Mast Road
Manchester, NH 03102
(603) 669-3270

NEW JERSEY DIVISION, INC.
CN2201
North Brunswick, NJ 08902
(201) 297-8000

NEW MEXICO DIVISION, INC.
5800 Lomas Boulevard, N.E.
Albuquerque, NM 87110
(505) 262-1727

NEW YORK STATE DIVISION,
INC.
6725 Lyons Street
P.O. Box 7
East Syracuse, NY 13057
(315) 437-7025

LONG ISLAND DIVISION, INC.
535 Broad Hollow Road
(Route 110)
Melville, NY 11747
(516) 420-1111

NEW YORK CITY DIVISION, INC
19 West 56th Street
New York, NY 10019
(212) 586-8700

QUEENS DIVISION, INC.
111-15 Queens Boulevard
Forest Hills, NY 11375
(212) 263-2224

WESTCHESTER DIVISION, INC.
246 North Central Avenue
Hartsdale, NY 10530
(914) 949-4800

NORTH CAROLINA DIVISION,
INC.
222 North Person Street
P.O. Box 27624
Raleigh, NC 27611
(919) 834-8463

NORTH DAKOTA DIVISION,
INC.
Hotel Graver Annex Building
115 Roberts Street
P.O. Box 426
Fargo, ND 58102
(701) 232-1385

OHIO DIVISION, INC.
453 Lincoln Building
1367 Sixth Street
Cleveland, OH 44114
(216) 771-6700

OKLAHOMA DIVISION, INC.
1312 N.W. 24th Street
Oklahoma City, OK 73106
(405) 525-3515

OREGON DIVISION, INC.
910 N.E. Union Avenue
Portland, Oregon 97232
(503) 231-5100

PENNSYLVANIA DIVISION, INC.
Route 422 & Sipe Avenue
P.O. Box 416
Hershey, PA 17033
(717) 533-6144

PHILADELPHIA DIVISION, INC.
21 South 12th Street
Philadelphia, PA 19107
(215) 665-2900

PUERTO RICO DIVISION, INC.
(Avenue Domenech 273
Hato Rey, PR)
GPO Box 6004
San Juan, PR 00936
(809) 764-2295

RHODE ISLAND DIVISION, INC.
345 Blackstone Boulevard
Providence, RI 02906
(401) 831-6970

SOUTH CAROLINA DIVISION,
INC.
2442 Devine Street
Columbia, SC 29205
(803) 256-0245

SOUTH DAKOTA DIVISION, INC.
1025 North Minnesota Avenue
Hillcrest Plaza
Sioux Falls, SD 57104
(605) 336-0897

TENNESSEE DIVISION, INC.
2519 White Avenue
Nashville, TN 37204
(615) 383-1710

TEXAS DIVISION, INC.
3834 Spicewood Springs Road
P.O. Box 9863
Austin, TX 78766
(512) 345-4560

UTAH DIVISION, INC.
610 East South Temple
Salt Lake City, UT 84102
(801) 322-0431

VERMONT DIVISION, INC.
13 Loomis Street, Drawer C

Montpelier, VT 05602
(802) 223-2348

VIRGINIA DIVISION, INC.
3218 West Cary Street
P.O. Box 7288
Richmond, VA 23221
(804) 359-0208

WASHINGTON DIVISION, INC.
2120 First Avenue North
Seattle, WA 98109
(206) 283-1152

WEST VIRGINIA DIVISION, INC.
Suite 100
240 Capital Street
Charleston, WV 25301
(340) 344-3611

WISCONSIN DIVISION, INC.
611 North Sherman Avenue
P.O. Box 1626
Madison, WI 53701
(608) 249-0487

MILWAUKEE DIVISION, INC.
6401 West Capital Drive
Milwaukee, WI 53216
(414) 461-1100

WYOMING DIVISION, INC.
Indian Hills Center
506 Shoshoni
Cheyenne, WY 82001
(307) 638-3331

AFFILIATE OF THE
    AMERICAN CANCER SOCIETY
Canal Zone Cancer Committee
Drawer A
Balboa Heights, CZ 00101

# National and regional education and self-help organizations

The following is a list of groups that have been formed to meet specific needs of people with cancer and their families. This list contains support groups, self-help groups, and organizations created to help people with rehabilitation.

*Corporate Angel Network:* Arranges free transportation (regardless of ability to pay) to and from treatments for cancer patients and one family member on planes of corporations who have volunteered space. Must be ambulatory (crutches and wheelchairs accepted). Call (914) 328-1313.

*Leukemia Society of America, Inc.:* This group provides financial assistance and consultation services for referral to other local support groups for people with leukemia and allied disorders. For more information about the program and local chapters, contact: Leukemia Society of America, Inc., 211 East 43 Street, New York, NY 10017 (210) 573-8484.

*Make Today Count:* Make Today Count brings together seriously ill people and concerned members of the community to discuss and resolve personal and emotional problems. The organization is for emotional self-help only and does not become involved in the medical or financial aspects of cancer. For more information, contact: Make Today Count, P.O. Box 303, Burlington, IA 52601 (319) 754-7266 or (319) 754-8977.

*United Cancer Council, Inc.:* The UCC is a federation of voluntary cancer agencies which seeks to control cancer through a three-point program of service, education, and research. Agencies are funded through the United Way in most communities where they are located. For further information on this national voluntary agency, contact: United Cancer Council, Inc., 1803 North Meridian Street, Indianapolis, IN 46202 (317) 923-6490.

*United Ostomy Association:* This nonprofit organization is made up of ostomates whose goal is providing mutual aid, moral support, and education to those who have had colostomy, ileostomy, or ureterostomy surgery. This association has several publications that are very helpful: For more information, contact: United Ostomy Association, Inc., 2001 West Beverly Boulevard, Los Angeles, CA 90057 (213) 413-5510.

*CanSurmount:* The goals of the CanSurmount program are: to provide carefully selected and trained volunteers or cancer patients to visit with other cancer patients and their families; to furnish continuing education and support for volunteers; to provide cancer patients and their families with current information which enables them to cope with the disease more effectively; to help health professionals to better understand the needs of cancer patients and their families; and to help the public understand those needs. For further information, contact: The American Cancer Society, 777 Third Avenue, New York, NY 10017 (212) 371-2900.

*Reach to Recovery:* This program provides rehabilitation support for women who have had mastectomies by meeting their physical, psychological, and cosmetic needs. The program works through a core of carefully trained volunteers who have successfully adjusted to their own surgery. For further information, contact your local office of the American Cancer Society.

*International Association of Laryngectomies:* This is an umbrella organization of 255 local clubs that promote and support the total rehabilitation of people with laryngectomies.

*The National Foundation for Ileitis and Colitis, Inc.,* 295 Madison Avenue, New York, NY 10017 (212) 685-3440.

*The National Hospice Organization:* An organization of hospice health care facilities providing help for the terminally ill and their families. For further information, contact: National Hospice Organization, 1311A Dolley Madison Boulevard, McLean, VA 22101 (703) 356-6770.

*National Self-Help Clearing House:* Repository for information on various support groups which deal with medical, health, emotional, and family problems. Individuals outside New York City are referred to local self-help clearinghouses. NYC residents can receive information on starting local support groups as well as a referral to existing local groups. For information, contact: National Self-Help Clearing House, C.U.N.Y. Graduate Center, 33 West 42d Street, New York, NY 10036 (212) 840-7606.
   The following programs offer support services to those residing in the immediate area:

*Cancer Call-PAC (People Against Cancer):* A telephone service which offers emotional support to people with cancer and their families. For information, contact: Service and Rehabilitation Director, The American Cancer Society, Illinois Division, 37 South Wabash Avenue, Chicago, IL 60603 (302) 372-0471.

*UCLA Psychological Telephone Counseling Service:* Free counseling directed to the psychosocial needs of people with cancer and care-givers. Monday through Friday, 9–5. Calls from area codes other than 213, 714, and 805 can call toll-free (800-352-7422). For further information, contact: U.C.L.A. Comprehensive Cancer Center, 1100 Glendon Avenue, Suite 844, Los Angeles, CA 90024 (213) 824-6017.

*Cancer Care, Inc., the National Cancer Foundation:* This voluntary social service agency provides professional counseling and planning to advanced cancer patients and their families. Plans for nursing care, homemakers, home-health aides, housekeepers, and other services are arranged. Direct services are provided primarily in the tri-state metropolitan region of New York, New Jersey, and Connecticut. For more information, contact: Cancer Care, Inc., One Park Avenue, New York, NY 10016 (212) 679-5700.

*TOUCH (Today Our Understanding of Cancer Is Hope):* A rehabilitation service co-sponsored by the Alabama Division of The American Cancer Society and the Comprehensive Cancer Center at the University of Alabama in Birmingham. For information, contact: Coordinator, Cancer Control Program, the University of Alabama, Birmingham, 104 Old Hillman Building, University Station, Birmingham, AL 35294 (205) 934-2620.

# Nutrition information centers

Massachusetts Nutrition Resource
  Center
(Nutrition Hot Line)
600 Washington Street
Boston, MA 02111
(617) 727-7173
Monday–Friday, 10 AM–2 PM
After 2:00 PM you may leave a
  message

Nutrition Information and
  Resource Center
Benedict House
Pennsylvania State University
University Park, PA 16802

(814) 865-6323
Monday–Friday, 8 AM–5 PM

The Nutrition Information Center
A component of the Clinical Nutri-
  tion Research Unit
The New York Hospital-Cornell
  Medical Center
Memorial Sloan-Kettering Cancer
  Center
515 East 71st Street, S-904
New York, NY 10021
(212) 472-6958
Monday–Friday, 9 AM–5 PM

# Pain control referral groups

Committee on Pain Therapy and
  Acupuncture
American Society of
  Anesthesiologists
515 Busse Highway
Park Ridge, IL 60068
(312) 825-5586

International Association for the
  Study of Pain
Department of Anesthesiology

Room RN-10
Univeristy of Washington
School of Medicine
Seattle, WA 98195
(206) 292-7521

National Hospice Organization
1311-A Dolley Madison Boulevard
McLean, VA 22101
(703) 356-6770

# Pain clinics, a partial listing

CALIFORNIA
Theresa Brechner, M.D., Director
U.C.L.A. School of Medicine
Department of Anesthesiology
Los Angeles, California
(213) 824-6241

Margo McCaffery, R.N.
Pain Specialist
Santa Monica, California
(213) 828-7251

B. Millman, M.D., Director
Stanford University School of
  Medicine
Department of Anesthesiology
Stanford, California
(415) 497-6238

FLORIDA
H. Rosonoff, M.D., Director
University of Miami Medical
  School

Department of Neurosurgery
Miami, Florida
(305) 547-6946

MASSACHUSETTS
G. Aranoff, M.D., Director
Boston Pain Center
Massachusetts Rehabilitation
    Hospital
Boston, Massachusetts
(617) 523-1818

NORTH CAROLINA
B. Nashold, M.D., Director
B. Urban, M.D., Director
Duke Medical Center
Durham, North Carolina
(919) 684-6255

NEW JERSEY
C. Ballinger, M.D., Director
Martland Hospital
Department of Anesthesiology
Newark, New Jersey
(201) 643-9012 Ext. 2827
(201) 643-8800 Ext. 2481

NEW YORK
K. Foley, M.D., Director
Memorial Sloan-Kettering Cancer
    Center

Pain Clinic
New York, New York
(212) 794-7050

B. Wolff, M.D., Director
Comprehensive Pain Center
New York University
New York, New York
(212) 340-6620

R. Kanner, M.D., Director
Albert Einstein College of
    Medicine
Pain Clinic
New York, New York
(212) 430-2833

TEXAS
Charles Kemp, M.D., Director
Home Hospice Program
Dallas, Texas
(214) 369-5500

WASHINGTON
J. Bonica, M.D., Director
University of Washington Pain
    Clinic
School of Medicine
Seattle, Washington
(206) 543-2672

# Childhood Cancer Programs

*Candlelighters:* A national organization formed by parents of children with cancer. Family support groups under the auspices of Candlelighters have many functions: exchanging practical information on ways of dealing with common problems; providing an outlet for frustrations through informal self-help sessions; offering a social outlet for parents and siblings to reduce the sense of isolation often imposed by cancer; disseminating information through meetings featuring medical speakers, psychologists, and other professionals; and directing families to professional counseling, if desired. For more information on Candlelighters chapters and programs, contact: Candlelighters Foundation, 123 C Street, S.E., Washington, DC 20003 (202) 483-9100, (202) 544-1696.

*Ronald McDonald Houses:* Ronald McDonald Houses provide lodging at economical rates for families of seriously ill children. Houses are located in Philadelphia, Chicago, Denver and twenty-nine other cities nationwide and thirty-six additional cities are committed to opening houses in the near future. For further information contact: Mr. A. L. Jones, Ronald McDonald House Coordinator, c/o Golin Communications, Inc. 500 N. Michigan Avenue, Chicago, IL 60611 (312) 836-7100.

Your local American Cancer Society may have information about other organizations in your vicinity which can help you either financially, emotionally, or through rehabilitation programs.

## Publications from the National Cancer Institute

The following list available from the National Cancer Institute focuses mainly on publications that deal with nutrition. However, the Institute publishes a wide range of material written on all aspects of cancer.

All National Cancer Institute publications are available free-of-charge. Allow at least 4 to 6 weeks for delivery.

A complete list of NCI publications can be obtained by writing or calling:

Publications Order
Office of Cancer Communications
National Cancer Institute
9000 Rockville Pike
Building 31, Room 10A18
Bethesda, MD 20205
(301) 496-5583

*"Cancer Treatment" Medicine for the Layman Series* (80-1807). Pamphlet describes cell growth in normal and in cancerous tissues; treatment with surgery, radiation, and chemicals; and how drugs are developed and how they work. A question-and-answer section is included.

*"Frontiers of Cancer Research, A Report to the People: 1979"* (81-2219). Illustrated booklet describes ongoing research activities at the National Cancer Institute and recounts progress in the prevention, treatment, and control of cancer. Includes a glossary of terms.

*"If You've Thought About Breast Cancer."* Pamphlet contains information about symptoms of breast cancer, detection, diagnosis, treatment, rehabilitation, breast reconstruction, and other information helpful to patients and their families.

*"Progress Against Breast Cancer, What You Can Do About It"* (81-1621). Leaflet summarizes current information about breast cancer, including detection, treatment, and rehabilitation.

*"Progress Against . . ."* (Series). This series contains information on causes, symptoms, diagnosis, treatment, and research in various cancer sites.

Cancer of the Bladder (81-722)  Cancer of the Mouth (81-118)
Cancer of the Bone (81-721)  Cancer of the Skin (81-310)
Hodgkin's Disease (81-172)  Cancer of the Testis (79-1492)
Cancer of the Larynx (81-448)  Cancer of the Uterus (79-171)
Leukemias, Lymphomas & Multi-
   ple Myeloma (81-329)

*"Research Reports" (Series).* In-depth reports covering current research on the cause and prevention, symptoms, detection, diagnosis, and treatment of various types of cancer.

*"Science and Cancer"* (80-568). Paperback book presents the medical and biological aspects of cancer as a practical problem. Its 20 chapters range over a wide field of subjects: diagnosis and treatment, nutrition and cancer, and anticancer drugs. (Of special interest to high school science teachers and students.)

*"Breast Reconstruction: Creating a New Breast Contour After Mastectomy"* (81-2151). Leaflet discusses techniques used in breast reconstruction, advantages and disadvantages of the procedure, types of implants used, how to choose a plastic surgeon, possible complications, and other factors concerned with breast reconstruction. Includes illustrations and a glossary.

*"Chemotherapy and You: A Guide to Self-Help During Treatment"* (81-1136). A booklet in question-and-answer format which addresses problems and concerns of patients receiving chemotherapy. Emphasis is on explanation, self-help, and participation during treatment. Includes glossary of terms and appendices on frequently used anticancer drugs.

*"Diet and Nutrition: A Resource for Parents of Children with Cancer"* (81-2038). Contains information about the importance of nutrition, side effects of cancer and cancer treatment, ways to encourage your child to eat, and special diets.

*"Eating Hints: Recipes and Tips for Better Nutrition During Cancer Treatment"* (81-2079). Originally produced by the Yale-New Haven Medical Center and reprinted by the NCI. A cookbook-style booklet. Includes recipes and tips for maintaining optimum but realistic nutrition during treatment. All recipes have been tested.

*"If You've Had Breast Cancer"* (81-2400). Leaflet offers suggestions on follow-up care for mastectomy patients, including recommendations for patients with lymphedema. Contains a glossary of terms and a listing of toll-free telephone numbers of cancer information offices.

*"Radiation Therapy and You: A Guide to Self-Help During Treatment"* (80-2227). This booklet, a cooperative venture between the NCI and the Michigan Cancer Foundation/Henry Ford Hospital, addresses problems and concerns of patients receiving radiation therapy. Emphasis is on explanation, self-help, and patient participation during treament. It is written in question-and-answer format and includes glossary of terms.

*Solving the Eating Problems of Cancer Patients.* B. L. Johnson; M. E. Morra; N. Suski. 1979. Free book. A survey of 99 cancer patients helped to determine the contents of this book, which includes many hints for increasing the enjoyment of eating, in addition to basic nutritional information for patients undergoing treatment. Emphasis is placed on adapting the patient's usual food preferences to new nutritional needs and to the special eating problems of a cancer patient—specifically those of nausea and vomiting; loss of appetite; mouth soreness and dryness; fatigue; intestinal upset; lactose intolerance; and the need for low-fat, low-sugar, and low-sodium or high-protein diets.

*"Taking Time: Support for People with Cancer and the People Who Care About Them"* (80-2059). A well-written booklet for people with cancer and their families. It addresses the feelings and concerns of others in similar situations and tells how they have coped.

*"The Leukemic Child"* (81-863). The mother of a leukemic child tells her story and gives advice for other parents in the same situation.

*"What You Need to Know About Cancer . . ."* (Series). This series of pamphlets designed for cancer patients discusses symptoms, diagnosis, rehabilitation, emotional issues, and questions to ask the doctor. Includes glossary of terms and Cancer Information Service telephone numbers.

Cancer (General) (79-1566)
Bladder (81-1559)
Bone (81-1571)
Brain and Spinal Cord (81-1558)
Breast (81-1588)
Colon and Rectum (78-1552)
Dysplasia, Very Early Cancer and
    Invasive Cancer of the Cervix
    (81-2047)
Esophagus (80-1557)
Hodgkin's Disease (81-1555)
Kidney (81-1569)
Larynx (81-1568)
Leukemia, Adult (80-1572)
Leukemia, Childhood (81-1573)

Lung (79-1553)
Melanoma (81-1563)
Mouth (80-1574)
Multiple Myeloma (80-1575)
Non-Hodgkin's Lymphoma (81-
    1567)
Ovary (81-1561)
Pancreas (81-1560)
Prostate (81-1576)
Skin (81-1564)
Stomach (81-1554)
Testis (81-1565)
Uterus (80-1562)
Wilms' Tumor (81-1570)

# Other materials related to cancer and nutrition

## BOOKS

*Health Through Nutrition: A Comprehensive Guide for the Cancer Patient.* E. H. Rosenbaum; C. A. Stitt; H. Drasin; I. R. Rosenbaum. 1978. $6.95

» *Alchemy Books*
  *681 Market Street, Suite 755,*
  *San Francisco, CA 94105.*
  *(415) 362-2708*

*You Can Fight Cancer and Win.* J. E. Brody and A. I. Holleg. 1977. $12.50 hard-cover, $4.95 paperback

» *In your bookstore or*
*New York Times Books*
*3 Park Avenue*
*New York, NY 10016*
*(212) 725-2050*


*Choices.* M. Morra and E. Pohs. 1980, $8.95

Presents a variety of approaches to eating and maintaining weight. Stresses the active role you can play in alleviating nutritional problems before they become severe. Special diets and recipes are given.

» *In your bookstore or*
*Avon Books*
*224 West 57th Street*
*New York, NY 10019*
*(212) 262-8871*


*Something's Got to Taste Good: The Cancer Patient's Cookbook.* J. Fishman, B. Anrod, 1981. $6.95

Creative, easy recipes with protein and calorie infomation given for each recipe. Included are suggestions for increasing protein and calorie levels and protein calorie tables of common foods and fast foods.

» *In your bookstore or*
*Andrews & McMeel Publishing Co.*
*1271 Avenue of the Americas*
*New York, NY 10020*
*(212) 582-0650*


*A Guide to Good Nutrition During and After Chemotherapy and Radiation.* S. Aker; P. Lenssen. 2d ed., 1979. $3.50

A guide to choosing easily tolerated foods to gain or maintain weight. Based on the experiences and suggestions of other patients, guidelines are presented to determine recommended calorie and protein intake. Separate sections cover easy, high-calorie, high-protein recipes, ideas for making food more appetizing, and commercially available nutritional supplements.

» *Fred Hutchinson Cancer Research Center,*
*1124 Columbia Street*
*Seattle, WA 98104*
*(206) 292-6301*


## PAMPHLETS

"Nutrition: A Helpful Ally in Cancer Therapy." Free

A summary of good nutrition and weight maintenance for cancer patients. Discusses ways in which the disease and various treatments can interfere with nutrition. Suggestions are provided for dealing with loss of appetite, nausea, diarrhea, constipation, dryness of the mouth, and early satiety. Information is given on boosting calorie and protein intake and using commercially prepared supplements.

» *Ross Laboratories*
  *Columbus, OH 43216*
  *Order No. G543*

"Blenderized Diet." J. Kukachka. Free
Emphasizes nutritionally balanced meals that are appealing in taste, smell, and color. Hints are given for blending, freezing, liquefying, and seasoning various foods. A typical daily menu and recipes for high-protein main dishes and desserts are included.

» *University of Wisconsin*
  *Clinical Cancer Center*
  *Public Affairs Office*
  *1900 University Avenue*
  *Madison, WI 53705*
  *(608) 262-0046*

"Esophagostomy or Pharyngostomy Tube Feeding." M. L. Olson. Free
Discusses preparation and administration of liquid food, along with common problems such as the addition of medications to food when esophageal or pharyngeal tube feeding is necessary.

» *Marian Olson, R.N.*
  *Department of Head and Neck Surgery and Oncology*
  *Roswell Park Memorial Institute,*
  *666 Elm Street*
  *Buffalo, NY 14263*
  *(716) 845-3278*

"High Protein Soft Diet." University of Wisconsin Clinical Cancer Center. Free
A diet developed to provide adequate nutrient intake for those who have difficulty swallowing following radiotherapy.

» *University of Wisconsin*
  *Clinical Cancer Center*
  *Public Affairs Office*
  *1900 University Avenue*
  *Madison, WI 53705*
  *(608) 262-0046*

"Home Care Guide for Patients With Head and Neck Disease." Wisconsin Head and Neck Network. Free
Self-care for patients who are tube feeding following tracheotomy, laryngectomy, or other head and neck surgery. Toma and wound care, sectioning, and oral hygiene are discussed.

» *University of Wisconsin*
*Clinical Cancer Center*
*Public Affairs Office*
*1900 University Avenue*
*Madison, WI 53705*
*(608) 262-0046*

"Looking Forward ... A Guidebook for the Laryngectomee." R. L. Keith; H. C. Shane; H. L. C. Coates; K. D. Devine. 1977. $1.25 plus postage and handling
Illustrated handbook features various aspects of self-care for laryngectomy patients, including tube feeding and instructions for preparation of liquid diets.

» *Schmidt Printing, Inc.*
*1416 Valley High Drive N.W.*
*Rochester, MN 55901*

"Diseases of the Colon and Rectum." American Medical Association. $.50

» *American Medical Association*
*Order Department OP-367*
*535 North Deerborn Street*
*Chicago, IL 60601*

"Naso-Gastric Tube Feeding." M. L. Olson. Free
Instructions are given for food preparation, introduction of liquid food via the naso-gastric tube, and management of routine problems.

» *Marian Olson, R.N.*
*Department of Head and Neck Surgery and Oncology*
*Roswell Park Memorial Institute*
*666 Elm Street*
*Buffalo, NY 14263*
*(716) 845-3278*

"Nutrition and the Oncology Patient." July 1979.
An explanation of the nutritional problems experienced during radiation or chemotherapy. Methods of controlling symptoms that interfere with eating, such as dry mouth, mouth blindness, and nausea, are covered. Additional information is included on improving taste and increasing nutritional value in food preparation.

» *Shands Teaching Hospital and Clinics*
*Department of Food and Nutrition Services*
*University of Florida*
*Gainesville, FL 32610*
*(904) 392-3575*

"Oro-gastric Tube Feeding." M. L. Olson. Free
A guide to home care outlining instructions for preparing liquid foods, methods for administering food, and management of common side effects.

» *Marian Olson, R.N.*
*Department of Head and Neck Surgery and Oncology*
*Roswell Park Memorial Institute*
*666 Elm Street*
*Buffalo, NY 14263*
*(716) 845-3278*

"Progressive Blenderized Diet." $.50

Information for those who need liquid or soft diets. Nutrition, meal patterns, commercial supplements, and food preparation (including seasoning) are covered. The blenderized diets and suggested meal patterns are arranged progressively—from liquid tube feedings to modified full liquid, purée soft, mechanical soft, and soft.

» *Shands Teaching Hospital and Clinics*
*Department of Food and Nutrition Services*
*University of Florida*
*Gainesville, FL 32610*
*(904) 392-3575*

"Restricted Fiber Diet." University of Wisconsin Clinical Cancer Center. Free

Diet designed to decrease the amount of bulk in the bowel. It specifies the protein, vitamins, minerals, and other nutrients needed to maintain good health.

» *University of Wisconsin*
*Clinical Cancer Center*
*Public Affairs Office*
*1900 University Avenue*
*Madison, WI 53705*
*(608) 262-0046*

"Soft and Blended Foods (for Head and Neck Radiation Patients)." C. Persigehl, comp. Revised 1976. $1.25

Recipes and sample menus for high-protein soft diets are suggested for patients undergoing head and neck radiation therapy. Lists of recommended foods and names of commercial high-protein formulas are provided.

» *Department of Patient and Family Support*
*151 East Bannock*
*Boise, ID 83702*
*(208) 386-2760*

"Chemotherapy: Your Weapon Against Cancer." M. E. Kulkin; E. M. Greenspan. 1978. $2

Explains chemotherapy's actions against cancer, explores its benefits and risks, and answers many questions about the process. Tips on nutritional needs are covered, as well as possible gastrointestinal side effects.

» *The Chemotherapy Foundation*
*2 East 86th Street*
*New York, NY 10028*
*(212) 988-2986*

"Nutrition for Patients Receiving Chemotherapy and Radiation Treatment." American Cancer Society. Free

Recipes for high-protein beverages, snacks, and desserts are featured. The preparation of liquid formulas for oral, tube, and nasal feeding is described; and sample menus, information on diet supplements, and a brief bibliography are included.

» *American Cancer Society, local units.*

"Nutritional Guide for Patients Receiving Upper and Lower Abdominal Radiation Therapy." C. Persigehl, comp. $1.75

Lists foods recommended or disallowed for restricted-residue diets. Ways of increasing the protein and caloric content of the diet are explained, and names of commercial diet supplements are listed. High-protein, nutritionally balanced sample menus are provided, along with suggestions for making the foods attractive and palatable, controlling diarrhea, and coping with nausea and vomiting.

» *Department of Patient and Family Support*
*151 East Bannock*
*Boise, ID 83702*
*(208) 386-2760*

"On Nutrition and Liquid Diet." M. L. Olson. Free

Describes methods of preparing liquid food for at-home tube feedings. Instructions are given for converting components from the major food groups into a liquid form, for storing liquid foods prepared in bulk, and for preparing meals with all food components blended into a single fluid. Information on caloric and nutritional content and on commercially available liquid foods is also supplied.

» *Marian Olson, R.N.*
*Department of Head and Neck Surgery and Oncology*
*Roswell Park Memorial Institute*
*666 Elm Street*
*Buffalo, NY 14263*
*(716) 845-3278*

"A Diet Guide for Chemotherapy Patients." Ellis Fischel State Cancer Hospital. Free

Diet is recommended for patients undergoing chemotherapy. Emphasis is on a high-protein diet and ample fluid intake. Gives tips to maintain appetite and prevent or control diarrhea.

» *Ellis Fischel State Cancer Hospital*
*Business 70 and Garth Avenue*
*Columbia, MO 65201*
*(314) 449-2711*

"Food for Those Who Hesitate . . . Tips that They Might Tolerate." J. E. Helsel. $.40

Offers diet and nutrition tips and selected recipes for patients undergoing chemotherapy. Recommendations are given for (1) the size and timing of meals, (2) the kinds of foods that are easy to swallow or tolerate, and (3) ways to increase protein and caloric intake.

» *Duke University Comprehensive Cancer Center*
*Cancer Information Services*
*P.O. Box 2985*
*Durham, NC 27710*
*(919) 684-3895*

"Nutrition During and After Radiation Therapy and Chemotherapy." S. M. Williams. 1978 Free

Basic eating guidelines are suggested; and tips for dealing with nausea, sore mouth, and other adverse effects from treatment are offered.

» *Hospital of the Good Samaritan*
*Oncology-Hematology Department*
*616 South Witmer Street*
*Los Angeles, CA 90017*
*(213) 488-8123*

"Radiation Therapy: How It Can Help You." L. Chilton. Free

Describes the nature and procedures of radiation therapy. Information about follow-up visits, diet, and recommended activities during therapy is provided.

» *National Cancer Institute*
*Office of Cancer Communications*
*9000 Rockville Pike*
*Building 31 Room 10A18*
*Bethesda, Maryland 20205*
*(800) 638-6694*

"Dietary Tips for Possible Nutrition-Related Problems in the Pediatric Cancer Patient." K. Moore. 1978. $1

Offers dietary tips to counteract such problems as nausea, anorexia, dehydration, and the adverse effects of chemotherapy drugs. Some high calorie recipes, especially appealing to children, are provided.

» *Kristina Moore, R.D.*
*1165 Eureka Avenue*
*Los Altos, CA 94022*
*(415) 968-9888*

"Nutrition Concerns . . . for Troubled Eaters During Radiation Therapy to the Head and Neck Areas." Memorial Sloan-Kettering Cancer Center. 1981. $3

Offers nutrition, diet, and recipe tips for persons undergoing radiation therapy. Information on tube feeding and tube feeding formulas are given. Answers frequently asked questions.

» *Memorial Sloan-Kettering Cancer*
   *Center, Food Service Department*
*1275 York Avenue, New York, NY 10021*
*(212) 794-7071*

# Low-sodium information

Sources of additional information on low-sodium diets and low-sodium recipes available at your local bookstore:

*Cooking Without Your Salt Shaker.* American Heart Association. David McKay, 1980.

*Cooking Without A Grain of Salt.* Elma W. Bagg. Doubleday, 1964.

*Living With High Blood Pressure: The Hypertension Diet Cookbook.* J. D. Margie and J. C. Hunt. Chilton Book Company, 1978.

*Secrets of Salt-Free Cooking.* Jeanne Jones. 101 Productions, 1979.

The American Heart Association also has booklets geared to specific sodium levels—500, 1,000, and 2,000 milligrams. These booklets are available (free of charge) only if they are ordered by your physician. Have your doctor order them through the local chapter of the American Heart Association or from: American Heart Association, 7320 Greenvillle Avenue, Dallas, TX 75231.

# *10*

## APPETIZERS, BEVERAGES,

## AND SNACKS

CHEESE BALL · CHEESE SPREAD · SPICY ROASTED PECANS · GRANOLA · MUSHROOM AND CHEESE APPETIZERS · TEX-MEX DIP · CURRY DIP · ZIPPY DIP · MEXICAN DIP · CURRIED CANTALOUPE DIP · TURKEY NIBBLERS · GREEK FETA CHEESE TRIANGLES · JELLY SNACK · APPLESAUCE TOAST · CRANBERRY BANANA TOAST · APPLE CHEESE SNACK · GRANOLA BARS · SNACK PACKS · ZESTY OYSTER CRACKERS · ORANGE SQUARES · CRISP TOAST · BREAKFAST IN A GLASS · BREAKFAST SHAKE · MEAL IN A GLASS · ORANGE EGGNOG · STRAWBERRY-BANANA YOGURT COOLER · BLENDER BANANA · TROPIC FIZZ · WINTER WARMER · GLOW WINE · ELEGANT ICED COFFEE · CRANBERRY COCKTAIL · SPARKLING APPLE CIDER · TANGY FRUIT JUICE COCKTAIL · TART TROPICAL FIZZ · FLOATING RAINBOW · APPLE-LIME COOLER · CRANBERRY DELIGHT

# CHEESE BALL

*Keep in the refrigerator for a cheese-and-cracker snack.*

1 package (8 ounces) cream cheese, softened
4 ounces blue cheese
1 cup shredded sharp Cheddar cheese (4 ounces)

1 small onion, minced
1 tablespoon Worcestershire sauce
$\frac{1}{2}$ cup chopped pecans

Mix all ingredients thoroughly. Store in covered container in refrigerator.

About $2\frac{1}{2}$ cups      2 tablespoons = 110 calories
                                        4 gm protein

# CHEESE SPREAD

2 packages (3 ounces each) cream cheese, softened
8 ounces blue cheese
2 cups shredded sharp Cheddar cheese (8 ounces)
$\frac{1}{2}$ cup white wine

$\frac{1}{2}$ cup sherry
1 teaspoon Worcestershire sauce
2 tablespoons grated onion
Dash each salt, garlic powder, and pepper sauce

Soften cream cheese and blue cheese in bowl with fork. Blend in Cheddar cheese. Stir in remaining ingredients and beat until smooth. Store in covered containers in refrigerator.

5 cups      $\frac{1}{4}$ cup = 130 calories
                          6 gm protein

# SPICY ROASTED PECANS

*Eat a handful for a zippy snack.*

2 packages ($12\frac{1}{2}$ ounces each) pecan halves
2 tablespoons plus $1\frac{1}{2}$ teaspoons margarine or butter, melted

$\frac{1}{3}$ cup Worcestershire sauce
2 to 3 drops pepper sauce
Coarse salt and freshly ground pepper

Heat oven to 325°. Spread pecan halves in baking pan, 13 × 9 × 2 inches. Mix margarine, Worcestershire sauce, and pepper sauce; pour over nuts and toss until nuts are coated. Bake about 25 minutes, shaking pan once or twice during baking, until nuts are lightly colored and sizzling. Sprinkle salt and pepper over nuts and shake pan to distribute seasonings. Cool nuts. Store in airtight containers in refrigerator.

About 3 cups  $\frac{1}{4}$ cup = 250 calories
3 gm protein

## GRANOLA

4 cups rolled oats
$\frac{1}{3}$ cup brown sugar (packed)
$\frac{1}{2}$ cup wheat germ
$\frac{1}{2}$ cup coconut

$\frac{1}{4}$ cup sesame seed
$\frac{1}{3}$ cup vegetable oil
$\frac{1}{4}$ cup honey
1 teaspoon vanilla

Heat oven to 350°. Spread rolled oats in baking pan, 13 × 9 × 2 inches. Heat in oven 10 minutes. Remove from oven; stir in sugar, wheat germ, coconut, and sesame seed. Mix oil, honey, and vanilla. Pour into pan and stir until dry ingredients are well coated. Bake 20 to 25 minutes, stirring mixture frequently. Cool. Stir until crumbly. Store in tightly covered container.

6 cups  $\frac{1}{2}$ cup = 250 calories
6 gm protein

## MUSHROOM AND CHEESE APPETIZERS

6 slices sandwich bread
Margarine or butter, melted
1 package (8 ounces) cream cheese, softened
$\frac{1}{4}$ cup margarine or butter, softened

2 egg yolks
1 teaspoon grated onion
1 can (6 ounces) sliced mushrooms, drained
Dash each salt and pepper sauce

Set oven control at broil or 550°. Remove crusts from bread slices; cut each slice into 4 squares or cut with a shaped cutter. Lightly brush one side of sections with melted margarine, and place on baking sheet. Toast 4 inches from heat until golden brown on buttered side.

Mix cream cheese, $\frac{1}{4}$ cup margarine, the egg yolks, and onion until smooth. Stir in mushrooms, and season with salt and pepper sauce. Spread on untoasted side of squares. Broil 4 inches from heat until topping is brown and bubbly. Serve hot.

24 appetizers  1 appetizer = 65 calories
1 gm protein

NOTE: Appetizers can be prepared up to the broiling step 4 to 6 hours before serving. Cover and refrigerate until ready to broil.

# TEX-MEX DIP

1 can (10½ ounces) plain or jala-
  peno-flavored bean dip
2 ripe small avocados
1 tablespoon lemon juice
¼ teaspoon salt
⅛ teaspoon pepper
½ cup dairy sour cream
¼ cup mayonnaise or salad dressing
½ package (¼ to 1⅛-ounce size) taco
  seasoning mix

½ cup chopped green onion with
  tops
1 cup chopped, seeded, peeled
  tomatoes
1 can (3½ ounces) pitted ripe olives,
  drained and chopped
1 cup shredded sharp Cheddar
  Cheese (about 4 ounces)
Large round tortilla chips

Spread bean dip into a 4 to 5-inch circle on serving plate. Remove peel and pits from avocados. Mash avocados with lemon juice, salt, and pepper until smooth. Spread mixture on cirlce of dip. Blend sour cream, mayonnaise, and taco seasoning mix; spread on avocado layer. Sprinkle layer each of onion, tomato, and olives; cover with cheese. Serve at room temperature with chips.

8 servings     Serving (7 ounces) = 35 calories
                           .8 gm protein

# CURRY DIP

*Prepare a day ahead.*

1 cup mayonnaise
1 teaspoon curry powder
¾ teaspoon celery seed
2 teaspoons Worcestershire sauce
1½ teaspoons lemon juice

⅛ teaspoon garlic powder
1 small onion, grated
1 teaspoon prepared mustard
1 teaspoon horseradish

Mix all ingredients, cover, and refrigerate 24 hours. Serve with carrot sticks, cauliflowerets, broccoli spears, and other favorite raw vegetables.

1 cup dip     2 tablespoons = 200 calories
                         ½ gm protein

# ZIPPY DIP

1 package (8 ounces) cream cheese,
   softened
1 tablespoon horseradish
½ teaspoon prepared mustard
1 teaspoon Worcestershire sauce

10 drops red pepper sauce
3 tablespoons pickle relish
3 tablespoons chili sauce
1 tablespoon lemon juice

Mix all ingredients until smooth. If thinner consistency is desired, mix in a small amount of milk.

About 1 cup     2 tablespoons = 115 calories
                                2 gm protein


# MEXICAN DIP

1 pound processed American
   cheese spread
1 can (16 ounces) tomatoes, drained
   and chopped

1 can (4 ounces) green chilies,
   drained and chopped
1 tablespoon instant minced onion
Corn or tortilla chips

Combine cheese spread, tomatoes, chilies, and onion in saucepan. Cook over low heat, stirring frequently, until cheese spread is melted. Pour into heatproof container and serve hot with corn chips.

3 cups     2 tablespoons = 60 calories
                            3 gm protein


# CURRIED CANTALOUPE DIP

1 large cantaloupe
1 carton (16 ounces) dairy sour
   cream
2 tablespoons mayonnaise
¼ to ½ teaspoon curry powder

1 teaspoon catsup
1 teaspoon minced onion
½ teaspoon salt
Dash pepper

Cut cantaloupe in half. Remove seeds and scoop out fruit with melon ball cutter. Run curved knife around inside of melon shells to make smooth. Turn melon shells upside down to drain. Return balls to shells. Mix remaining ingredients and pour over balls. Refrigerate. Serve with wooden picks.

About 24 melon balls     2 melon balls = 110 calories
                                      1 gm protein

# TURKEY NIBBLERS

1 cup minced cooked turkey  
½ cup mayonnaise  
¼ cup grated Parmesan cheese

½ teaspoon poultry seasoning  
24 slices cocktail bread  
Parsley sprigs

Mix turkey, mayonnaise, cheese, and poultry seasoning. Spread on bread slices. Place slices on baking sheet.

Set oven control at broil or 550°. Broil slices 4 to 6 inches from heat about 1 minute or until hot. Garnish each with parsley sprig. Serve hot.

24 nibblers     1 nibble = 65 calories  
                            3 gm protein

# GREEK FETA CHEESE TRIANGLES

*Freeze and save for a quick snack.*

1 package (17¼ ounces) frozen puff  
    pastry  
¾ pound feta cheese, crumbled

2 eggs  
¼ cup snipped parsley

Thaw pastry 20 minutes. Mix cheese, eggs, and parsley thoroughly. Unfold one pastry sheet; roll into rectangle, 12 × 9 inches, on lightly floured surface. Cut into 3-inch squares. Place 1 tablespoon cheese mixture in center of each square; moisten edges with water and fold pastry to form triangle. Press edges firmly together with fork to seal. Repeat with remaining pastry sheet and cheese mixture. Chill.

Heat oven to 425°. Bake on ungreased baking sheet 8 to 10 minutes, until puffed and golden brown. Serve warm.

24 triangles     1 triangle = 55 calories  
                            3 gm protein

NOTE: Unbaked triangles can be wrapped securely in plastic wrap and frozen until ready to bake. It is not necessary to thaw before baking.

# JELLY SNACK

*Don't eat your toast plain—add some calories.*

2 slices bread  
2 teaspoons margarine, softened

2 tablespoons your favorite jelly or  
    jam

Set oven control at broil or 550°. Toast bread slices on one side. Spread untoasted sides of bread with margarine, then spread each with 1 tablespoon jelly. Broil about 5 inches from heat until bubbly, about $\frac{1}{2}$ minute.

2 servings     1 slice = 210 calories
                        3 gm protein

## APPLESAUCE TOAST

*A quick and easy snack.*

$1\frac{1}{2}$ teaspoons butter or margarine,          Dash nutmeg
   melted                                Dash cinnamon
1 teaspoon sugar                                        2 slices bread
$\frac{1}{4}$ cup applesauce

Set oven control at broil or 550°. Mix margarine, sugar, applesauce, nutmeg, and cinnamon. Spread half of applesauce mixture to edges of each bread slice. Broil 5 inches from heat until hot and edges are light brown, 1 to 2 minutes. Watch closely. Optional: top toast with spoonful of sweetened whipped cream.

2 servings     1 slice = 120 calories
                        3 gm protein

NOTE: Applesauce mixture can be covered and stored in refrigerator.

## CRANBERRY BANANA TOAST

*A fancy toast for a teatime snack.*

1 slice bread                                   $\frac{1}{4}$ banana, sliced
1 teaspoon margarine, softened                  1 teaspoon brown sugar
1 tablespoon cranberry sauce                    $\frac{1}{4}$ teaspoon cinnamon

Set oven control at broil or 550°. Toast bread on one side. Spread untoasted side of bread with margarine, then with cranberry sauce. Arrange banana slices on cranberry sauce. Mix sugar and cinnamon; sprinkle on top. Broil about 5 inches from heat until bubbly, $\frac{1}{2}$ to 1 minute.

1 serving     1 slice = 158 calories
                       3 gm protein

### VARIATION
» Substitute $\frac{1}{4}$ teaspoon allspice or anise seed for the cinnamon.

# APPLE-CHEESE SNACK

4 large apples
2 cups shredded Cheddar cheese (8 ounces)

3 tablespoons Worcestershire sauce

Set oven control at broil or 550°. Core apples. Cut each apple into 4 slices; place on rack in broiler pan. Mix cheese and Worcestershire sauce; spread layer of cheese mixture on each apple slice. Broil 4 inches from heat 3 to 4 minutes, until cheese is melted. Serve hot as a snack, appetizer, or salad accompaniment.

16 slices    1 slice = 85 calories
                     4 gm protein


# GRANOLA BARS

*Keep on hand for a coffee break.*

3 cups 100% natural cereal
   (granola)
½ cup raisins
⅓ cup wheat germ

⅓ cup brown sugar (packed)
¼ cup margarine or butter
3 tablespoons honey

Heat oven to 350°. Line baking pan 9 × 9 × 2 inches with aluminum foil. Measure cereal, raisins, and wheat germ into large bowl. Heat sugar, margarine, and honey, stirring occasionally, until smooth. Pour over cereal mixture, mixing until it is well coated. Turn into pan. Bake 12 to 14 minutes, until golden brown. Cool. Remove from pan and remove foil. Cut into bars 2¼ × 1 inch.

36 bars    1 bar = 65 calories
                    1 gm protein

NOTE: Substitute ⅔ cup chopped nuts for the wheat germ.


# SNACK PACKS

*Carry a pack with you for a quick snack.*

5 cups honey graham cereal
1 cup salted peanuts
¼ cup creamy peanut butter

2 tablespoons margarine or butter
1 teaspoon cinnamon
1 cup raisins

Heat oven to 350°. Mix cereal and peanuts in large bowl. Heat peanut butter, margarine, and cinnamon in small saucepan over low heat, stirring occasionally, just until blended. Pour over cereal and peanuts, stirring until they are coated. Spread in ungreased baking pan, 13 × 9 × 2 inches. Bake 15 minutes, stirring occasionally. Stir in raisins; spread mixture on waxed paper, and let stand 2 hours. Pack ½ cup of mixture in each of 12 plastic sandwich bags. Store in a cool, dry place.

12 bags      1 bag = 200 calories
                          6 gm protein

# ZESTY OYSTER CRACKERS

1 cup oyster crackers                  Celery or onion salt
2 tablespoons margarine or butter

Melt margarine or butter in skillet. Add oyster crackers. Stir with fork or shake skillet to coat crackers on all sides. Sprinkle with celery or onion salt. Very good with tomato or chicken soup.

1 cup      ¼ cup = 100 calories
                        1 gm protein

# ORANGE SQUARES

4 slices bread                              2 tablespoons orange marmalade
2 tablespoons margarine or butter,   1 tablespoon margarine or butter,
   softened                                     softened

Heat oven to 400°. Trim crusts from bread slices. Spread bread slices with 2 tablespoons margarine. Spread 2 of the slices with marmalade and top each with a remaining bread slice. Brush tops with 1 tablespoon margarine. Place on ungreased baking sheet; cut each into 4 squares. Bake until brown and hot, about 8 minutes.

2 servings      1 square = 285 calories
                             4 gm protein

# CRISP TOAST

*If your taste sensation is decreased, try spicing up your toast.*

Set oven control at broil or 550°. Toast 4 slices bread 5 inches from heat 3 to 4 minutes on each side. Serve with one of the toppings below. Leftover toast can be wrapped in aluminum foil and frozen. Heat in toaster oven to crisp.

1 slice toast = 110 calories
                2 gm protein

### TOPPINGS

» *Garlic:* Mix 2 tablespoons margarine, softened, $\frac{1}{8}$ teaspoon garlic powder, and $\frac{1}{4}$ teaspoon marjoram.

» *Garlic Italian:* Mix 2 tablespoons margarine, softened, $\frac{1}{8}$ teaspoon garlic powder, and $\frac{1}{4}$ teaspoon oregano.

» *Parmesan:* Mix 2 tablespoons margarine or butter, softened, and 2 tablespoons Parmesan cheese.


# BREAKFAST IN A GLASS

1 medium banana
$\frac{1}{2}$ cup egg substitute
$\frac{1}{3}$ cup water
$1\frac{1}{2}$ tablespoons frozen orange juice
   concentrate (thawed)

1 teaspoon wheat germ
1 teaspoon honey
Dash salt

Slice banana into blender; add remaining ingredients. Blend on high speed until smooth, about 1 minute.

1 serving        1 serving = 370 calories
                            16 gm protein

NOTE: Egg substitutes are available in the frozen food or dairy section of your supermarket.


# BREAKFAST SHAKE

$\frac{3}{4}$ cup milk or half-and-half
$\frac{1}{4}$ cup egg substitute

1 banana, cut up
$\frac{1}{2}$ teaspoon vanilla

Place all ingredients in blender container. Cover and blend until smooth. Pour into large glass.

1 serving          1 serving = 315 calories
                               14 gm protein

VARIATIONS

» Substitute 1 peach (peeled, pitted, and cut up), 1 cup strawberries, or 1 cup blueberries for the banana.

NOTE: Egg substitutes are available in the frozen food or dairy section of your supermarket.

## MEAL IN A GLASS

*Blend any of the following combinations 5 to 10 seconds on high speed:*

1 cup milk
1 envelope (1.22 ounces) strawberry flavored instant breakfast drink
¼ cup crushed pineapple

1 serving = 320 calories
            15 gm protein

1 cup milk
1 envelope (1.22 ounces) vanilla flavored instant breakfast drink
¼ cup frozen raspberries, strawberries, or blueberries

1 serving = 345 calories
            15 gm protein

1 cup milk
1 envelope (1.22 ounces) vanilla flavored instant breakfast drink
1 jar (4½ ounces) pureed fruit (baby food) or 6 canned apricot halves

1 serving = 385 calories
            15 gm protein

1 cup milk
1 envelope (1.22 ounces) chocolate flavored instant breakfast drink
1 small banana, cut up

1 serving = 390 calories
            16 gm protein

## ORANGE EGGNOG

1 can (6 ounces) frozen orange juice concentrate (thawed)
2 cups half-and-half

2 cups commercial eggnog
Nutmeg

Blend orange juice and half-and-half until smooth. Stir in eggnog. Serve in glasses with a sprinkle of nutmeg and garnish with an orange slice if desired.

4 servings          1 serving (about 1¼ cups) = 120 calories
                                                 10 gm protein

# STRAWBERRY-BANANA YOGURT COOLER

½ cup plain yogurt       ½ banana
½ cup light cream (20%) or milk    ¼ cup egg substitute
½ cup strawberries      1 tablespoon sugar

Measure all ingredients into blender. Blend on high speed until smooth, about 30 seconds. Pour into tall glass.

1 serving      1 serving = 515 calories
                                  18 gm protein

NOTE: Egg substitutes are available in the frozen food or dairy section of your supermarket.


# BLENDER BANANA

1 cup light cream (20%)       1 small banana, cut up
1 tablespoon honey

Place all ingredients in blender. Blend on high speed until smooth, about 10 seconds. Serve immediately or freeze for a dessert.

1 serving      1 serving = 630 calories
                                  8 gm protein


# TROPIC FIZZ

4 scoops vanilla ice cream (about ½    1 bottle (10 ounces) carbonated
   pint)                                 orange-flavored drink
¼ cup drained crushed pineapple    Flaked coconut
¼ cup papaya nectar             Orange slices
                                   Fresh mint leaves

Mix 1 scoop ice cream, 2 tablespoons pineapple, and 2 tablespoons nectar in each of two 10-ounce glasses. Fill glasses with carbonated drink. Top each with scoop of ice cream, and sprinkle with coconut. Garnish with mint leaves and orange slices on wooden picks.

2 servings      1 serving (½ recipe) = 370 calories
                                         6 gm protein

# WINTER WARMER

1 bottle (25 ounces) claret wine
$\frac{3}{4}$ cup sugar

Peel of 2 oranges (cut with vegetable parer)
$\frac{1}{4}$ teaspoon cinnamon

Heat all ingredients, stirring until sugar is dissolved, just to simmering. Serve hot.

5 servings     1 serving ($\frac{2}{3}$ cup) = 230 calories
0 protein

# GLOW WINE

1 bottle (25 ounces) claret wine
$\frac{1}{2}$ cup plus 2 tablespoons sugar

$\frac{1}{4}$ cinnamon stick
1 whole clove

Heat all ingredients, stirring until sugar is dissolved, just to simmering. Remove spices before pouring. Serve hot.

5 servings     1 serving ($\frac{2}{3}$ cup) = 210 calories
0 protein

# ELEGANT ICED COFFEE

Crushed ice
6 cups cold double-strength coffee
$\frac{1}{2}$ cup whipping cream

$\frac{1}{2}$ cup sugar
2 tablespoons cognac, optional

Fill 6 tall glasses with crushed ice and place in freezer.

Measure 3 cups of the coffee, $\frac{1}{4}$ cup each of the cream and sugar, and 1 tablespoon cognac into blender. Blend on high speed about 15 seconds. Divide among 3 of the ice-filled glasses. Repeat with remaining ingredients for the remaining 3 glasses. Serve with straws.

6 servings     1 glass = 150 calories
1 gm protein

# CRANBERRY COCKTAIL

1 cup cranberry cocktail
¾ cup lemonade

½ bottle (7 ounces, scant ½ cup) ginger ale, chilled

Mix cranberry cocktail, lemonade, and ginger ale. Serve in glasses with ice cubes or crushed ice.

2 servings      1 cup = 140 calories
                        0 protein


# SPARKLING APPLE CIDER

*Double the calories of apple juice.*

1¼ cups apple juice
¼ cup fresh orange juice
2 thin slices unpared lime, quartered

1 thin slice unpared orange, quartered
4 ounces ginger ale, chilled

Combine apple juice, orange juice, and fruit pieces and refrigerate. At serving time, add ginger ale.

2 servings      1 serving (1 cup) = 105 calories
                        0 protein


# TANGY FRUIT JUICE COCKTAIL

⅓ cup water
⅓ cup sugar
1½ cups grapefruit juice

¾ cup pineapple juice
½ cup lime juice
Mint leaves

Heat water and sugar to boiling, stirring until sugar is dissolved. Cool.

Mix sugar and water and juices. Pour into chilled glasses and garnish with mint leaves.

4 servings      1 serving (¾ cup) = 135 calories
                        1 gm protein

NOTE: Sugar water and juices can be mixed in blender.

# TART TROPICAL FIZZ

1 cup grapefruit juice, chilled
½ cup orange juice, chilled
¼ cup pineapple juice, chilled

¾ cup club soda, chilled
1 cup lime sherbet
Mint leaves

Mix fruit juices and club soda. Serve in glasses with ice cubes or crushed ice and top each serving with a scoop of lime sherbet. Garnish with mint leaves.

2 servings    1 serving (1 cup) = 230 calories
                                   2 gm protein

NOTE: If you do not have fresh mint, substitute a thin slice of orange, lemon, or lime.


# FLOATING RAINBOW

1 cup orange juice
1 cup cranberry cocktail
1 cup unsweetened pineapple juice

2 bottles (20 ounces each) ginger
  ale, chilled
Mint leaves

Pour each fruit juice into refrigerator tray; freeze to make 12 cubes of each juice.
    To serve, place 3 cubes of each juice in each of 4 tall glasses; pour about ½ bottle ginger ale into each. Serve with colored straws.

4 servings    1 glass = 260 calories
                        1 gm protein

NOTE: Flavors develop as juice cubes melt.


# APPLE-LIME COOLER

½ pint lime ice

¾ cup apple juice, chilled

Soften lime ice. Stir in apple juice gradually until mixture is smooth. Pour into chilled glasses. Nice served with stick cinnamon stirrers.

2 servings    1 cup = 190 calories
                      1 gm protein

*Appetizers, Beverages, and Snacks*

# CRANBERRY DELIGHT

*A cool, calorie-packed refresher.*

1 cup cranberry juice
$\frac{1}{4}$ cup orange juice

1 cup vanilla ice cream, slightly
   softened

Measure all ingredients into blender container. Cover and blend until smooth. Pour into glasses and serve with straws.

2 servings     1 glass = 230 calories
                         3 gm protein

# 11

## SOUPS, SALADS, SANDWICHES

TOPPERS FOR SOUPS · BONUS POTATO SOUP · EASY NEW ENGLAND CLAM CHOWDER . CRABMEAT SOUP · CREAM OF SPINACH SOUP · HEARTY VEGETABLE SOUP · CREAMY PEA SOUP · CHILLED POTATO SOUP   COLD CREAM OF AVOCADO SOUP · EASY CHILLED SOUPS · VICHYSSOISE · COLD CUCUMBER SOUP · CHILLED CHICKEN AVOCADO SOUP · FIESTA SALAD · ZIPPY APPLE SALAD · TUNA-MUSHROOM-MACARONI SALAD · CONFETTI SALAD · CRUNCHY CHICKEN SALAD · EGG AND ASPARAGUS SALAD   CRANBERRY SALAD · MEAL ON A MUFFIN · HAWAIIAN TOAST SANDWICH · EGG SALAD SANDWICH   HOT SEAFOOD SANDWICHES · TOASTY TURKEYWICHES · SLOPPY JOE · QUICK PIZZA (WITH MEAT) · QUICK PIZZA (NO MEAT) · PIZZA PICK-UPS · PEPPERONI PIZZA · OPEN-FACED SALMON SANDWICH · FRUIT 'N' TUNA SANDWICH · BEEF AND MUSHROOM SANDWICH ·

## TOPPERS FOR SOUPS

*Green Pea Soup*

Beat $\frac{1}{4}$ cup whipping cream until stiff; stir in $\frac{1}{2}$ teaspoon horseradish.

*For Beef Broth or Tomato Soup*

Beat $\frac{1}{4}$ cup whipping cream; stir in $\frac{1}{4}$ teaspoon minced onion.

*For Jellied Consommé*

Beat $\frac{1}{4}$ cup whipping cream until stiff; stir in 1 teaspoon grated lime peel and $\frac{1}{2}$ teaspoon sherry.

Each makes enough for 6 to 8 servings.

## BONUS POTATO SOUP

$\frac{1}{2}$ cup chopped celery
1 tablespoon butter or margarine
1 can (10$\frac{1}{2}$ ounces) condensed
  potato soup

1 soup can milk or light cream
  (20%)
1 can (5 ounces) boned chicken or
  turkey, cut up
1 tablespoon snipped parsley

Cook and stir celery in margarine until tender. Stir in remaining ingredients; heat, stirring constantly, just to simmering. Reduce heat and simmer about 5 minutes.

$3\frac{1}{2}$ cups      1 cup = 230 calories
                        13 gm protein

## EASY NEW ENGLAND CLAM CHOWDER

1 can (7 or 8 ounces) minced clams
$\frac{1}{4}$ cup chopped onion
2 tablespoons margarine or butter

1 cup diced pared potato
2 cups light cream (20%) or milk
Salt and pepper

Drain clams, reserving liquid. Cook and stir onion in margarine until tender. Stir in potato and reserved clam liquid. Heat to boiling. Reduce heat, cover, and cook until potato is tender. Stir in clams and cream. Heat just to simmering, stirring constantly. Reduce heat and simmer about 10 minutes, stirring occasionally. Season with salt and pepper.

4 cups      1 cup = 190 calories
                    9 gm protein

# CRABMEAT SOUP

1 package (6 ounces) frozen cooked
    crabmeat, thawed
1 pint half-and-half

1 can (10½ ounces) chicken broth
2 tablespoons sherry, optional
Salt and white pepper

Drain crabmeat and remove cartilage. Heat half-and-half to boiling in top of double boiler over hot water. Stir in broth, crabmeat, and sherry; continue cooking until heated through. Season with salt and white pepper. Serve in warm bowls. If desired, soup can be refrigerated and served cold.

4 cups      1 cup = 235 calories
                    12 gm protein


## CREAM OF SPINACH SOUP

2 packages (10 ounces each) frozen
    chopped spinach, thawed
2 cans (10½ ounces each) condensed
    cream of chicken soup

2 small onions, cut up
2 soup cans light cream (20%)
¼ cup snipped parsley

Drain spinach. Combine spinach, soup, and onion in blender; mix on high speed until smooth. Pour into saucepan; stir in cream and heat, stirring constantly, just to simmering. Reduce heat and simmer 5 minutes, stirring frequently. Serve in cups or bowls, topped with parsley.

8 cups      1 cup = 250 calories
                   6 gm protein


## HEARTY VEGETABLE SOUP

1 pound ground beef
⅔ cup chopped onion
1 can (46 ounces) tomato juice
2 cans (16 ounces) mixed
    vegetables

2 beef bouillon cubes
1 teaspoon seasoned salt
1 teaspoon sugar

Cook and stir meat and onion in large saucepan until meat is brown and onion is tender. Stir in remaining ingredients. Heat to boiling. Reduce heat, and simmer 30 minutes, stirring occasionally.

9 cups      1 cup = 165 calories
                 16 gm protein

# CREAMY PEA SOUP

1 can (11¼ ounces) condensed green pea soup
1 can (10½ ounces) condensed cream of potato soup

2 soup cans milk or light cream (20%)
⅛ teaspoon thyme leaves, crushed
Dash nutmeg

Heat all ingredients in large saucepan, stirring constantly, just to simmering. Reduce heat and simmer about 10 minutes, stirring frequently.

5½ cups        1 cup = 205 calories
                        9 gm protein

# CHILLED POTATO SOUP

1 can (10½ ounces) condensed cream of potato soup
1 soup can light cream (20%) or milk

½ cup dairy sour cream
¼ cup finely chopped cucumber

Heat soup, cream, sour cream, and cucumber, stirring constantly, just to simmering. Pour into blender; blend on high speed until smooth. Cover and refrigerate 4 hours. Serve in chilled bowls.

3 cups        1 cup = 215 calories
                      5 gm protein

# COLD CREAM OF AVOCADO SOUP

3 medium to large avocados
Few drops onion juice
2 cups chicken consommé
1 cup dairy sour cream

1 cup light cream (20%)
Salt and freshly ground pepper
Paprika

Slice avocados into blender. Add onion juice and consommé. Blend on high speed until smooth. Add sour cream and cream and blend on low speed 5 seconds. Season with salt and pepper. Cover and refrigerate at least 4 hours. Serve in chilled mugs or bowls with a sprinkle of paprika.

8 cups        1 cup = 265 calories
                      4 gm protein

## EASY CHILLED SOUPS

These condensed soups are excellent served cold:

Bisque of tomato
Black bean
Consommé (chill to jell; do not add liquid)
Cream of asparagus
Cream of celery
Cream of chicken
Green pea
Tomato

Mix soup with water, milk, or light cream (20%), and refrigerate about 4 hours. To save time, keep cans of soup in refrigerator; then mix with cold water, milk, or light cream (20%). Using milk or cream instead of water will add extra protein and calories.

## VICHYSSOISE

1 can (10$\frac{1}{2}$ ounces) condensed cream of potato soup
1 soup can light cream (20%) or milk
Snipped chives or parsley

Heat soup and cream, stirring constantly, just to simmering. Pour into blender; blend on high speed until smooth. Cover and refrigerate at least 4 hours. Serve in chilled bowls. Sprinkle chives on top.

2$\frac{3}{4}$ cups     1 cup = 140 calories
                       4 gm protein

## COLD CUCUMBER SOUP

1 can (10$\frac{1}{2}$ ounces) condensed cream of celery soup
1 cup milk
1 small cucumber, cut up
Dash pepper sauce
Dash salt and pepper
1 cup dairy sour cream

Blend soup, milk, cucumber, pepper sauce, and seasonings in blender on high speed until smooth. On low speed, blend in sour cream. Cover and refrigerate at least 4 hours. Serve in chilled bowls.

3$\frac{1}{2}$ cups     1 cup = 265 calories
                       6 gm protein

*Soups, Salads, Sandwiches*

# CHILLED CHICKEN AVOCADO SOUP

1 can (10½ ounces) condensed cream
   of chicken soup
1 soup can light cream (20%)

½ cup chopped celery
1 to 2 tablespoons chopped onion
1 ripe avocado

Blend soup, cream, celery, and onion in blender on high speed until smooth. Cover and refrigerate at least 4 hours.
   Slice avocado into blender with soup; blend on high speed until smooth. Serve in chilled mugs or bowls.

4 cups      1 cup = 320 calories
                    5 gm protein


# FIESTA SALAD

*A change-of-pace side dish packed with nutrition.*

1 package (7¼ ounces) macaroni and
   cheese dinner
1 cup chopped tomato
½ cup chopped cucumber

½ cup shredded carrot
½ cup salad dressing
¼ teaspoon salt
⅓ cup shredded Cheddar cheese

Cook macaroni and cheese dinner as directed on package. Turn into bowl; add remaining ingredients and toss. Chill for 1 hour.

4 servings     1 serving (about 1 cup) = 290 calories
                              7 gm protein


# ZIPPY APPLE SALAD

*If your taste is dulled, this should perk it up.*

⅓ cup cooked pasta
1 cup diced unpared tart apple
   (about 1 medium)

¼ cup mayonnaise
¼ teaspoon horseradish
2 lettuce leaves

Combine pasta and apple. Mix mayonnaise and horseradish; pour on pasta and apple and toss. Cover and refrigerate. Serve on lettuce.

2 servings     1 serving (¾ cup) = 262 calories
                          1 gm protein

» *Apple Salad with Pomegranate Seed:* Add 1 teaspoon pomegranate seeds before tossing salad.

» *Apple-Grape Salad:* Add 10 seedless green grapes or seeded halved red grapes before tossing salad.

» *Apple-Celery Salad:* Add 1 tablespoon diced celery before tossing salad.

# TUNA-MUSHROOM-MACARONI SALAD

1 package (8 ounces) elbow
 macaroni
8 ounces mushrooms
2 teaspoons lemon juice
¼ cup thinly sliced scallion greens

3 tablespoons olive oil
½ teaspoon salt
¼ teaspoon thyme
1 can (7 ounces) tuna, drained
8 to 10 pitted ripe olives, sliced

Cook macaroni as directed on package. Slice mushrooms into bowl; drizzle with lemon juice and toss until moistened. Add scallion greens, oil, salt, and thyme and toss. Stir in macaroni, tuna, and olive slices. Refrigerate about 1 hour.

4 to 6 servings   1 serving (⅕ recipe) = 250 calories
18 gm protein

# CONFETTI SALAD

*Cool and delicious.*

1 can (15½ ounces) pineapple
 chunks, drained (reserve syrup)
1½ cups diced cooked ham
1 cup cubed Cheddar cheese

2 oranges, pared and sectioned
Lettuce
⅓ cup mayonnaise
⅓ cup dairy sour cream

Combine pineapple chunks, ham, cheese, and orange sections, and toss. Refrigerate at least 1 hour.

Turn salad into lettuce-lined serving bowl. Mix mayonnaise, sour cream, and reserved syrup; serve in small bowl accompanying salad.

4 servings   1 serving (about 1⅓ cups) = 600 calories
21 gm protein

*Soups, Salads, Sandwiches*

# CRUNCHY CHICKEN SALAD

4 cups diced cooked chicken
1 cup chopped celery
1 cup halved seedless green grapes
1 cup slivered almonds, toasted
1 teaspoon salt

$\frac{1}{4}$ teaspoon pepper
$\frac{3}{4}$ cup mayonnaise
$\frac{1}{4}$ cup dairy sour cream
Lettuce

Combine chicken, celery, grape halves, and almond slivers in bowl. Mix salt, pepper, mayonnaise, and sour cream; pour over chicken mixture and toss. Cover and refrigerate about 2 hours. Serve on lettuce.

6 servings     1 serving ($1\frac{1}{2}$ cups) = 520 calories
                                         34 gm protein

# EGG AND ASPARAGUS SALAD

6 hard-cooked eggs, separated
2 tablespoons vegetable oil
1 tablespoon vinegar
1 tablespoon mayonnaise
Dash freshly ground pepper

1 pound asparagus, cooked,
    drained, and cooled; or 1 can (16
    ounces) asparagus spears,
    drained
1 tablespoon grated orange peel
$\frac{2}{3}$ cup French dressing

Mash egg yolks with fork. Mix in oil, vinegar, mayonnaise, and pepper until smooth. Chop egg whites; stir into egg yolk mixture. Mound egg mixture in center of serving platter. Arrange asparagus spears around egg mixture and sprinkle the spears with orange peel. Serve with French dressing.

4 servings     1 serving ($\frac{1}{4}$ recipe) = 400 calories
                                         12 gm protein

# CRANBERRY SALAD

*A tart gelatin salad.*

1 can (8 ounces) crushed pineapple
1 package (3 ounces) strawberry-
    flavored gelatin
$\frac{1}{3}$ cup mayonnaise
$\frac{1}{4}$ teaspoon salt

2 tablespoons vinegar
1 can (6 ounces) evaporated milk
1 can (16 ounces) whole cranberry
    sauce
Lettuce leaves

Drain pineapple, reserving juice. Measure juice and add water to make $\frac{3}{4}$ cup. Heat liquid to boiling. Stir in gelatin until dissolved. Cool.

Mix mayonnaise, salt, and vinegar; blend in gelatin mixture. Stir in milk, pineapple, and cranberry sauce. Pour into 4-cup mold. Refrigerate until firm. Unmold onto lettuce-lined serving plate. Top with sour cream.

6 to 8 servings    1 serving (about $\frac{1}{2}$ cup) = 265 calories
3 gm protein

## MEAL ON A MUFFIN

$\frac{1}{2}$ cup chopped onion
1 medium green pepper, diced
$\frac{1}{4}$ cup margarine or butter
$\frac{1}{8}$ teaspoon salt
Dash pepper

4 eggs
1 can ($4\frac{1}{2}$ ounces) roast beef or ham spread
2 English muffins, split and toasted

Cook and stir onion and green pepper in 1 tablespoon of the margarine until vegetables are crisp-tender. Season with salt and pepper. Melt remaining margarine in large skillet; fry eggs to desired consistency. Spread roast beef spread on muffin halves; top with egg and onion mixture.

4 muffin halves    $\frac{1}{2}$ muffin = 350 calories
18 gm protein

## HAWAIIAN TOAST SANDWICH

3 tablespoons margarine or butter, softened
1 teaspoon cinnamon
1 teaspoon curry powder
8 slices white bread

8 thin slices cooked ham (1 ounce each)
1 can ($8\frac{1}{4}$ ounces) sliced pineapple, drained
4 slices Swiss cheese (1 ounce each)

Mix margarine, cinnamon, and curry powder; spread mixture on one side of each slice of bread.

Set oven control at broil or 550°. Toast bread slices spread sides up on broiler rack 4 inches from heat until spread is light brown. Remove from oven; top each slice with 1 ham slice, $\frac{1}{2}$ pineapple slice, and $\frac{1}{2}$ cheese slice. Sprinkle cinnamon over top. Broil until cheese is melted and light brown. Serve immediately.

4 servings    1 sandwich = 530 calories
24 gm protein

# EGG SALAD SANDWICH

2 hard-cooked eggs, finely chopped
2 tablespoons mayonnaise
1 teaspoon chopped pimiento
$\frac{1}{4}$ teaspoon dry mustard

Salt and pepper to taste
2 slices bread
Lettuce leaf

Mix egg, mayonnaise, pimiento, and mustard. Season with salt and pepper, and spread on one slice bread. Top with lettuce leaf and remaining slice bread.

1 serving        1 sandwich = 470 calories
                                18 gm protein


# HOT SEAFOOD SANDWICHES

1 package (6 ounces) frozen crabmeat and/or shrimp, thawed
1 cup shredded Cheddar cheese (4
  ounces)
$\frac{1}{2}$ cup finely chopped celery
1 tablespoon snipped parsley
$\frac{1}{2}$ cup chopped ripe olives

$\frac{1}{4}$ cup mayonnaise or salad dressing
1 teaspoon lemon juice
$\frac{1}{2}$ teaspoon Dijon-style mustard
$\frac{1}{2}$ teaspoon Worcestershire sauce
4 English muffins, split
$\frac{1}{4}$ cup margarine or butter

Drain crabmeat/shrimp. Combine seafood, cheese, celery, parsley, and olives in bowl. Mix mayonnaise, lemon juice, mustard, and Worcestershire sauce; pour over seafood mixture and toss.

Set oven control at broil or 550°. Toast muffin halves, and spread margarine on toasted side. Top each with about $\frac{1}{4}$ cup seafood mixture. Broil 4 inches from heat 4 to 5 minutes or until cheese topping is melted.

4 servings        1 sandwich = 425 calories
                                22 gm protein


# TOASTY TURKEYWICHES

2 cups diced cooked turkey
1 can (7 ounces) whole kernel corn,
  drained
$\frac{1}{2}$ cup chopped celery
$\frac{2}{3}$ cup salad dressing or mayonnaise
1 teaspoon prepared mustard

$\frac{1}{4}$ teaspoon salt
$\frac{1}{8}$ teaspoon pepper
16 slices bread
$\frac{1}{2}$ cup margarine or butter
8 slices process American cheese

Heat oven to 425°. Mix turkey, corn, celery, salad dressing, mustard, salt, and pepper. Spread bread slices on one side with margarine. Place 8 slices buttered side down on ungreased baking sheet. Top each with cheese slice, $\frac{1}{3}$ cup turkey mixture, and a remaining bread slice, buttered side up. Bake 6 to 8 minutes until brown. Turn and bake 2 to 3 minutes longer until second side is brown.

8 servings　　　1 sandwich = 535 calories
　　　　　　　　　　　23 gm protein

## SLOPPY JOE

1 pound ground lean beef
1 can (10$\frac{1}{2}$ ounces) condensed cream
　of mushroom soup
$\frac{1}{2}$ cup dairy sour cream
1 teaspoon horseradish, optional

$\frac{1}{4}$ cup chopped green pepper or
　pimiento
6 hamburger buns, split and
　toasted

Cook and stir ground beef in skillet until brown. Stir in soup, sour cream, horseradish, and green pepper. Heat, stirring constantly, just to simmering. Reduce heat, and simmer 10 to 15 minutes, stirring occasionally. Serve on buns.

6 servings　　　1 serving (1 bun with $\frac{1}{6}$ recipe) = 320 calories
　　　　　　　　　　　　　　22 gm protein

## QUICK PIZZA (WITH MEAT)

$\frac{1}{2}$ cup tomato juice
2 ounces cooked ground beef
1 tablespoon chopped green
　pepper
2 tablespoons chopped fresh
　mushroom
Dash garlic powder

Dash salt and pepper
$\frac{1}{8}$ teaspoon basil
$\frac{1}{4}$ teaspoon oregano
1 whole wheat English muffin,
　split and toasted
2 teaspoons margarine or butter
2 slices onion, separated into rings

Heat oven to 400°. In small saucepan, heat to boiling all ingredients except muffin, margarine, and onion, stirring occasionally. Reduce heat and simmer uncovered 5 minutes. Spread muffin halves with margarine, then spoon meat mixture onto each, and top with onion rings. Place on ungreased baking sheet and bake 3 minutes.

1 serving　　　1 pizza muffin = 340 calories
　　　　　　　　　25 gm protein

# QUICK PIZZA (NO MEAT)

1 whole wheat English muffin,
  split and toasted
2 teaspoons margarine or butter
1 tablespoon tomato paste
1 tablespoon water
1 tablespoon finely chopped green
  pepper

$\frac{1}{8}$ teaspoon basil
$\frac{1}{8}$ teaspoon oregano
Dash each garlic salt and pepper
$\frac{1}{2}$ cup shredded mozzarella cheese
$\frac{1}{2}$ teaspoon parsley flakes
2 thin onion rings
1 fresh mushroom, sliced

Heat oven to 400°. Spread toasted side of each muffin half with 1 teaspoon margarine. Mix remaining ingredients except parsley flakes, onion rings, and mushroom; spread on muffin halves. Sprinkle with $\frac{1}{2}$ cup shredded cheese and parsley flakes. Top each muffin half with an onion ring and mushroom slices. Place on ungreased baking sheet. Bake until bubbly, 3 to 5 minutes.

1 serving      1 pizza muffin = 375 calories
                              18 gm protein

# PIZZA PICK-UPS

*Can be frozen and reheated for a quick, easy meal.*

2 loaves frozen bread dough,
  thawed
$\frac{1}{2}$ pound ground lean beef
1 envelope ($1\frac{1}{2}$ ounces) spaghetti
  sauce mix

1 can (6 ounces) tomato paste
1 cup water
1 cup shredded mozzarella cheese
  (4 ounces)

Place frozen bread dough in refrigerator for 12 hours to thaw.

Cook and stir ground beef in skillet until brown. Stir in sauce mix, tomato paste, and water. Heat to boiling, stirring constantly. Reduce heat; simmer 10 minutes, stirring occasionally.

Heat oven to 400°. On floured surface, roll 1 loaf dough into rectangle, 16 × 8 inches. Spread half the meat sauce on dough. Sprinkle with half the cheese. Roll from long side as for jelly roll. Cut into 4 slices. Place on greased baking sheet. Repeat with remaining bread dough. Bake 15 to 20 minutes, until golden brown. Serve hot.

8 servings      1 pick-up = 370 calories
                           19 gm protein

# PEPPERONI PIZZA

*A flavorful mini-meal in minutes.*

2 tablespoons marinara sauce
2 Whole wheat English muffins,
   split and toasted

1 cup shredded mozzarella cheese
   (4 ounces)
16 thin slices pepperoni

Set oven control at broil or 550°. Spoon marinara sauce on each of 4 muffin halves. Top with layer of cheese and slices of pepperoni. Broil 4 inches from heat until cheese is melted.

2 servings     1 pizza muffin = 340 calories
                             20 gm protein


# OPEN-FACED SALMON SANDWICH

$\frac{1}{2}$ cup drained canned salmon
$1\frac{1}{2}$ teaspoons cranberry-orange
   relish
1 tablespoon mayonnaise

1 teaspoon chopped onion
2 slices bread
1 tablespoon snipped parsley

Mix salmon, relish, mayonnaise, and onion. Spread on bread slices; sprinkle with parsley.

2 servings     1 open-faced sandwich = 215 calories
                                 18 gm protein


# FRUIT 'N' TUNA SANDWICH

1 slice bread or 1 English muffin
   half
1 ounce drained tuna
2 tablespoons well-drained crushed
   pineapple

1 teaspoon lemon juice
$\frac{1}{4}$ teaspoon ginger
2 tablespoons mayonnaise

Set oven control at broil or 550°. Toast bread on 1 side (do not toast muffin). Mix tuna, pineapple, lemon juice, ginger, and mayonnaise with fork. Spread untoasted side of bread with tuna mixture. Broil 5 inches from heat until light brown, about 3 minutes.

1 serving     1 open-faced sandwich = 315 calories
                                 11 gm protein

# BEEF AND MUSHROOM SANDWICH

*Radishes add a bit to this mini-meal.*

1 slice bread
2 teaspoons margarine or butter
2 radishes, sliced
Salt and pepper to taste

2 ounces chopped cooked beef
$\frac{1}{4}$ cup beef gravy
$\frac{1}{4}$ cup sliced fresh or canned
  mushrooms

Spread bread with margarine and toast in oven. Arrange radish slices on toast. Heat remaining ingredients in small saucepan over low heat, just to simmering. Spoon beef mixture over radish slices. Serve hot and garnish with radish roses if desired.

1 serving     1 sandwich = 265 calories
                        22 gm protein

# *12*

## BREADS

EVER-READY MUFFINS · BANANA BREAD · HIGH-FIBER BREAD ·
CRANBERRY-BANANA BRAN BREAD · BEST BANANA NUT
BREAD · YOGURT-HONEY BREAD · ZUCCHINI BREAD ·
PUMPKIN NUT BREAD · BRAN BATTER BREAD · FRENCH
TOAST · FRENCH TOAST WITH MAPLE PECAN SYRUP ·
ORANGE FRENCH TOAST · HOT CEREAL · COTTAGE CHEESE
PANCAKES

# EVER-READY MUFFINS

*Wonderful for a high-fiber diet.*

3 cups unprocessed wheat bran
1 cup boiling water
1 cup brown sugar (packed)
½ cup vegetable oil or margarine
2 eggs, beaten

1½ cups whole-wheat flour
1 cup all-purpose flour
2½ teaspoons baking soda
1 teaspoon salt
2 cups milk

Measure 1 cup of wheat bran into large bowl. Pour boiling water over bran; cover and set aside to steep 5 minutes.

Stir in remaining wheat bran, sugar, oil, eggs, flours, soda, salt, and milk until blended. Pour batter into tightly covered plastic container(s) and store in refrigerator at least 12 hours before baking. (Batter will keep in refrigerator 6 weeks.)

To bake, heat oven to 400°. Grease desired number of muffin cups. Fill cups ½ full. Bake 18 to 20 minutes.

30 Muffins        1 muffin = 125 calories
                           3 gm protein

NOTE: For added calories and variation, divide batter and stir chopped apple (with red peel), chopped cranberries, dates, or raisins into different batches.

# BANANA BREAD

½ cup margarine or butter
¾ cup brown sugar (packed)
1 egg
1¼ cups mashed banana (3 medium)
¼ cup yogurt

1 cup all-purpose flour
1 cup whole-wheat flour
1 teaspoon baking powder
1 teaspoon baking soda
¼ teaspoon salt

Heat oven to 350°. Grease loaf pan 9 x 5 x 3 inches. Cream margarine and sugar in large bowl until fluffy. Stir in egg, banana, and yogurt. Blend in flours, baking powder, baking soda, and salt. Pour into pan. Bake 55 minutes or until wooden pick inserted in center comes out clean. Cool in pan 10 minutes. Remove and cool on rack.

1 loaf (about 12 slices)        1 slice = 165 calories
                                        3 gm protein

# HIGH-FIBER BREAD

*A mini-meal when served with a glass of milk.*

1 cup all-purpose flour
¾ cup whole-wheat flour
½ cup wheat germ
½ cup sugar
2 teaspoons baking powder
1 teaspoon salt
6 eggs
1 cup milk

¼ cup molasses
1 teaspoon vanilla
¼ cup margarine or butter, melted
2 cups fruit and fiber cereal with
   dates, raisins, walnuts
½ cup raisins
½ cup chopped walnuts

Heat oven to 350°. Grease loaf pan 9 x 5 x 3 inches. Mix flours, wheat germ, sugar, baking powder, and salt in large bowl. Beat eggs thoroughly. Beat in milk, molasses, and vanilla. Pour into bowl with flour mixture, and mix until blended. Stir in margarine, cereal, raisins, and nuts. Pour into pan. Bake 50 to 60 minutes or until wooden pick inserted in center comes out clean. Cool thoroughly. Wrap in aluminum foil and store at room temperature.

12 slices     1 slice = 290 calories
                    9 gm protein

# CRANBERRY-BANANA BRAN BREAD

*A tart quick-bread that makes an easy mini-meal.*

1 cup all-purpose flour
¾ cup whole-wheat flour
1 cup 100% bran cereal
⅔ cup sugar
2¾ teaspoons baking powder
½ teaspoon salt
⅓ cup margarine or butter

1 cup mashed ripe banana (2 to 3
   medium)
4 eggs, beaten
¼ cup milk
1 cup cranberries
1 cup chopped nuts

Heat oven to 350°. Grease loaf pan, 9 x 5 x 3 inches. Measure flours, cereal, sugar, baking powder, and salt into bowl. Cut in margarine thoroughly. Mix in banana, eggs, and milk, until just blended. Stir in cranberries and nuts.

Pour into pan. Bake 50 to 60 minutes or until wooden pick inserted in center comes out clean. Cool in pan 10 minutes. Remove from pan, and cool thoroughly before slicing.

12 slices     1 slice = 290 calories
                    7 gm protein

# BEST BANANA NUT BREAD

*Slice and freeze in portions for a quick snack.*

1½ cups mashed ripe banana (4 to 6 medium)
½ cup margarine, softened
1½ cups sugar
2 eggs
1 teaspoon vanilla
1 cup whole-wheat flour

1 cup all-purpose flour
½ cup bran flake cereal
1 teaspoon baking soda
1 teaspoon salt
½ cup buttermilk
1 cup chopped nuts
1 cup raisins

Heat oven to 350°. Grease 2 loaf pans 9 x 5 x 3 inches. Measure banana into large mixer bowl. Add margarine, sugar, eggs, and vanilla; beat at medium speed, scraping bowl frequently, until mixture is smooth and fluffy. Blend in flours, cereal, soda, salt, and buttermilk on low speed, scraping bowl occasionally. Stir in nuts and raisins.

Divide batter between 2 pans. Bake 60 minutes or until wooden pick inserted in center comes out clean. Cool in pan 10 minutes. Remove from pan and cool on wire rack.

2 loaves (about 12 slices each)     1 slice = 195 calories
3 gm protein


# YOGURT-HONEY BREAD

1 carton (16 ounces) plain yogurt
Juice of 1 lemon
3 eggs
½ cup honey

2½ cups whole-wheat flour
½ cup brown sugar (packed)
2½ teaspoons baking powder
½ teaspoon salt

Heat oven to 350°. Grease loaf pan 9 x 5 x 3 inches. Mix yogurt, lemon juice, eggs, and honey in large bowl. Mix in flour, sugar, baking powder, and salt. (Do not overmix.) Pour into pan. Bake 1 hour. Remove from pan and cool on rack.

12 slices     1 slice = 207 calories
7 gm protein

*Nutrition and the Cancer Patient*

# ZUCCHINI BREAD

2½ cups all-purpose flour
¼ cup nonfat dry milk
½ cup wheat germ
2 teaspoons baking soda
½ teaspoon baking powder
1 cup brown sugar (packed)
1 cup granulated sugar
3 teaspoons cinnamon

½ teaspoon nutmeg
1 cup vegetable oil
3 eggs
3 teaspoons vanilla
1½ cups chopped nuts
3 cups shredded unpared zucchini
  (about 4 medium)

Heat oven to 350°. Grease 2 loaf pans 9 x 5 x 3 inches. Measure all ingredients except nuts and zucchini into bowl; mix thoroughly. Stir in nuts and zucchini. Divide batter between pans. Bake 1 hour or until wooden pick inserted in center comes out clean.

2 loaves (about 12 slices each).      1 slice = 130 calories
                                                2 gm protein

VARIATION

» Substitute 1¼ cups whole-wheat flour for half the flour.


# PUMPKIN NUT BREAD

¼ cup margarine or butter
1 cup sugar
2 eggs
½ cup milk
1 cup mashed cooked pumpkin
2 cups all-purpose flour

2 teaspoons baking powder
½ teaspoon baking soda
1 teaspoon salt
1 teaspoon cinnamon
1½ teaspoons nutmeg
1 cup chopped nuts

Heat oven to 350°. Grease loaf pan 9 x 5 x 3 inches. Cream margarine and sugar in large bowl until fluffy. Stir in eggs, milk, and pumpkin. Blend in flour, baking powder, soda, salt, cinnamon, and nutmeg. Stir in nuts. Pour into pan. Bake 45 to 50 minutes or until wooden pick inserted in center comes out clean. Cool in pan 5 minutes. Remove and cool on rack.

12 slices      1 slice = 250 calories
                       5 gm protein

# BRAN BATTER BREAD

2¾ cups all-purpose flour  
2 teaspoons salt  
2 packages active dry yeast  
1¼ cups milk  

½ cup water  
3 tablespoons margarine or butter  
2 tablespoons honey  
2 cups bran cereal  

Combine the salt, yeast, and 1¼ cups of the flour in large mixer bowl. Heat milk, water, margarine, and honey over low heat to 120 to 130°. Stir in bran cereal. Pour into flour-yeast mixture. Beat at medium speed 2 minutes, scraping bowl occasionally. Add ¾ cup of the remaining flour; beat at high speed 2 minutes, scraping bowl frequently. Mix in remaining flour with spoon until smooth. Cover; let rise in warm place until double, 35 to 45 minutes.

Heat oven to 375°. Grease 1½-quart casserole. Stir down batter; beat vigorously about ½ minute. Pour into casserole. Bake 35 to 40 minutes or until loaf sounds hollow when lightly tapped. Remove from casserole and cool on rack. Excellent with honey butter.

12 slices    1 slice = 185 calories  
               6 gm protein


# FRENCH TOAST

*A crunchy version of an old favorite.*

8 slices white bread or French  
   bread  
2 eggs  
¼ cup orange juice  
¼ teaspoon salt  

½ cup cornflakes, crushed  
¼ cup wheat germ  
¼ cup ground nuts  
3 tablespoons margarine  

Trim crusts from bread slices, then cut each slice in half. In a flat bowl, beat eggs, orange juice, and salt with fork until blended. Mix cornflakes, wheat germ, and nuts in small pie pan or cake pan.

Heat margarine in large skillet. Dip bread slices into egg mixture, then in cornflake mixture, coating both sides. Place in skillet. Cook until brown on both sides, turning slices with broad spatula. Delectable served with confectioners' sugar or syrup.

4 servings    2 slices = 350 calories  
               12 gm protein

NOTE: To crush cornflakes, place in plastic bag, tie securely, and crush with hands.

# FRENCH TOAST WITH MAPLE PECAN SYRUP

2 eggs
½ cup milk
½ teaspoon salt
¼ teaspoon nutmeg
2 tablespoons margarine or butter

8 slices wheat berry bread or raisin
    bread
2 tablespoons chopped pecans
1 cup maple or pancake syrup

Beat eggs, milk, salt, and nutmeg in shallow bowl. Melt margarine in large skillet. Dip bread slices in egg mixture, coating both sides. Fry in skillet until brown, turning once. Stir nuts into syrup. Serve French toast with syrup mixture.

4 servings        2 slices = 440 calories
                           9 gm protein


# ORANGE FRENCH TOAST

2 eggs
⅓ cup orange juice
⅛ teaspoon cinnamon
2 tablespoons margarine or butter

4 slices day-old bread or thick
    slices French bread
Confectioners' sugar

Beat egg, orange juice, and cinnamon until fluffy. Melt margarine in skillet. Dip each bread slice into egg mixture to coat both sides; carefully transfer to skillet (do not crowd). Cook over medium heat until golden brown on both sides. Sprinkle with confectioners' sugar.

2 servings (2 slices each)        2 slices = 310 calories
                                          11 gm protein


## HOT CEREAL

Prepare your favorite hot cereal as directed on package, but add calories by substituting milk or cream for the water and stirring 2 tablespoons jam, jelly, marmalade, maple syrup, molasses, honey, or marshmallows into cereal.

Or, stir into hot cereal 1 to 2 tablespoons raisins, applesauce, mandarin orange segments, or cut-up apricots, dates, or prunes, and sprinkle brown sugar on top.

# COTTAGE CHEESE PANCAKES

3 eggs
1 cup cottage cheese

$\frac{1}{4}$ cup all-purpose flour
2 tablespoons vegetable oil

Beat eggs thoroughly. Add remaining ingredients, and beat until just blended. Drop batter by measuring tablespoonsful onto heated griddle. (If using electric griddle or frypan, heat to 300°.) Cook over medium-low heat until bubbles have broken; turn and cook until other side is golden. Even better served with applesauce.

Twelve 3-inch pancakes     1 pancake = 70 calories
                                             4 gm protein

NOTE: Leftover pancakes can be warmed in 350° oven.

# 13

## EGGS, CHEESE,
## PASTA, VEGETABLES

QUICK EGGS BENEDICT · EGG AND FRIES · SCRAMBLED EGGS · CHEESE AND ONION PIE · MACARONI AND CHEESE · OVEN MACARONI · BAKED SOUFFLE · CHEESE BAKE · SWISS FONDUE · BAKED CHEESE FONDUE · BASIC SOUFFLE · CHICKEN PUFF · CHEESE RAREBIT · CHICKEN QUICHE · QUICHE LORRAINE · CREOLE SAUCE OMELET ROLLS · MUSHROOM OMELET · OMELET AUX FINES HERBES · OMELET ROLL · MUSHROOM-SHRIMP SAUCE WITH OMELET ROLLS · CALIFORNIA SAUCE OMELET ROLLS · BAKED EGGS · CHEESY CREAMED EGGS · EGGS A LA KING · BAKED EGGS WITH CHEESE · OVEN SOUFFLE · COLD CURRIED EGGS · EGGS FOO YOUNG · BAKED EGGS PROVENCAL · SHIRRED EGGS WITH MUSHROOMS · EGGS BEARNAISE · BOB'S FAVORITE NOODLE CASSEROLE · FETTUCINI CARBONARA · HAM 'N' CHEESE PIE · HAM AND EGG EN CROUTE · BEST-EVER SPINACH · HAM AND MACARONI BAKE · EASY HAM AND MACARONI BAKE · CRISSCROSS POTATOES · CHEESE NOODLE CASSEROLE · SPINACH SUPREME

# QUICK EGGS BENEDICT

| | |
|---|---|
| 6 thin slices ham | $\frac{1}{3}$ cup milk |
| 2 tablespoons margarine or butter | 6 eggs |
| 1 can (10$\frac{1}{2}$ ounces) condensed cream of celery, chicken, or mushroom soup | 3 English muffins, split and toasted, or 6 slices bread, toasted |
| | 1 tablespoon snipped parsley |

Fry ham slices in margarine until light brown. Heat soup and milk, stirring constantly, just to simmering. Keep warm over low heat. Poach eggs.

Place 1 ham slice on cut side of each muffin half; top with poached egg, and spoon soup sauce on eggs. Garnish with parsley.

6 servings      1 serving = 410 calories
                            20 gm protein

# EGG AND FRIES

| | |
|---|---|
| 3 tablespoons margarine or butter | 4 eggs |
| 4 frozen hash-brown potato patties | Salt and pepper |

Melt margarine in skillet. Cook potato patties in skillet over medium heat 10 minutes. Turn patties; make a depression in each patty with back of spoon. Break an egg into each depression; season with salt and pepper. Cook over medium heat 5 to 6 minutes. Cover and cook 2 to 4 minutes to desired consistency.

4 servings      1 patty = 245 calories
                            7 gm protein

# SCRAMBLED EGGS

| | |
|---|---|
| 4 eggs | Dash pepper |
| 2 tablespoons cream | 1 tablespoon margarine or butter |
| $\frac{1}{4}$ teaspoon dry mustard | |

Mix eggs, cream, mustard, and pepper with fork, stirring thoroughly for a uniform yellow, or mixing just slightly if streaks of white and yellow are preferred.

Heat margarine in skillet over medium heat until just hot enough to sizzle a drop of water. Pour egg mixture into skillet. As mixture begins to set at bottom and side, gently lift cooked portions with spatula so the thin, uncooked portion can flow to bottom. Avoid constant stirring. Cook until eggs are thickened throughout but still moist, 3 to 5 minutes.

4 servings        1 serving ($\frac{1}{4}$ recipe) = 130 calories
                                    6 gm protein

NOTE: Substitute snipped chives, parsley, tarragon leaves, or chervil leaves for the dry mustard.

## CHEESE AND ONION PIE

Pastry for 9-inch one-crust pie or frozen pie shell
$\frac{3}{4}$ cup shredded sharp cheddar cheese (6 ounces)
1 tablespoon flour
1 large onion, cut into thin rings

2 tablespoons margarine or butter
1 cup milk
1 egg plus 1 egg yolk
$\frac{1}{2}$ teaspoon salt
$\frac{1}{8}$ teaspoon white pepper
Dash paprika

Heat oven to 400°. Prepare pastry. Toss cheese and flour in bowl. Cook onion rings in margarine until tender. In pastry-lined pie pan, layer half the onion rings, the cheese, and remaining onion rings. Beat milk, egg, egg yolk, salt, and pepper until blended; pour over layers. Sprinkle with paprika. Bake 15 minutes. Reduce oven temperature to 325°, and bake 25 to 30 minutes longer or until knife inserted in center comes out clean.

6 servings        $\frac{1}{6}$ pie = 390 calories
                             12gm protein

## MACARONI AND CHEESE

1 package (8 ounces) elbow macaroni
$\frac{1}{4}$ cup chopped onion
1 tablespoon margarine or butter

1 can (10$\frac{3}{4}$ ounces) condensed Cheddar cheese soup
$\frac{1}{2}$ cup milk
1 cup shredded Cheddar cheese

Cook macaroni as directed on package. Cook and stir onion in margarine until tender. Stir in soup, milk, and cheese, stirring constantly, until cheese is melted. Stir in macaroni and heat, stirring frequently, until bubbly.

4 to 6 servings        1 serving ($\frac{1}{5}$ recipe) = 330 calories
                                            13 gm protein

*Eggs, Cheese, Pasta, Vegetables*

# OVEN MACARONI

1 package (8 ounces) elbow
    macaroni
$\frac{1}{4}$ cup chopped onion
1 tablespoon margarine or butter
1 can (10$\frac{3}{4}$ ounces) condensed
    Cheddar cheese soup

$\frac{1}{2}$ cup light cream (20%)
1 cup shredded Cheddar cheese
1 tablespoon margarine or butter
2 tablespoons bread crumbs

Heat oven to 350°. Cook macaroni as directed on package. Turn into ungreased 1$\frac{1}{2}$-quart casserole. Cook and stir onion in 1 tablespoon margarine until tender. Stir in soup, cream, and cheese; pour over macaroni. Melt 1 tablespoon margarine; stir in bread crumbs. Sprinkle crumb mixture on casserole. Bake about 30 minutes, until bubbly and light brown.

4 servings    1 serving ($\frac{1}{4}$ recipe) = 490 calories
                        17 gm protein

# BAKED SOUFFLÉ

*A light mini-meal.*

1 tablespoon margarine or butter
1 egg
$\frac{1}{3}$ cup milk
$\frac{1}{3}$ cup dairy sour cream

$\frac{1}{8}$ teaspoon white pepper
$\frac{1}{2}$ small onion (about 2 inches in
    diameter), sliced

Heat oven to 325°. In oven, melt 1$\frac{1}{2}$ teaspoons margarine in each of two 10-ounce custard cups.

    Beat egg and milk with rotary beater. Mix in sour cream and pepper. Pour half the mixture into each custard cup. Top with onion slices. Bake uncovered until puffy and golden brown, about 40 minutes.

2 servings    1 serving (1 custard cup) = 210 calories
                        6 gm protein

# CHEESE BAKE

1 package (8 ounces) elbow
    macaroni
$\frac{1}{2}$ cup margarine or butter
2 tablespoons flour
1$\frac{1}{2}$ cups milk

1 teaspoon salt
$\frac{1}{4}$ teaspoon pepper
1 cup shredded process American
    cheese (4 ounces)
Paprika

Heat oven to 350°. Cook macaroni as directed on package. Melt margarine over low heat. Stir in flour. Cook over low heat, stirring constantly, until mixture is smooth and bubbly. Stir in milk, salt, and pepper. Heat to boiling, stirring constantly. Boil and stir 1 minute. Stir in macaroni. Turn into baking dish $11\frac{1}{2}$ x $7\frac{1}{2}$ x $1\frac{1}{2}$ inches. Sprinkle cheese over top and garnish with paprika. Bake 25 to 30 minutes, until cheese is melted.

4 to 6 servings      1 serving ($\frac{1}{5}$ recipe) = 470 calories
                                              14 gm protein

## SWISS FONDUE

*A slow, sociable meal.*

1 can (11 ounces) condensed Cheddar cheese soup
8 ounces natural Swiss cheese, cut into $\frac{1}{2}$ inch cubes
$\frac{1}{4}$ teaspoon prepared mustard

$\frac{1}{4}$ teaspoon Worcestershire sauce
$\frac{1}{4}$ teaspoon pepper sauce
French or Italian bread, cut into 1-inch cubes

Heat soup, cheese, mustard, Worcestershire sauce, and pepper sauce, stirring constantly, until cheese is melted. Pour into ceramic fondue pot; place over heat. Spear bread with fork and dip into hot cheese mixture. Citrus and apple sections make a tangy, crunchy accompaniment; the apple is good dipped, too.

4 servings      1 serving ($\frac{1}{4}$ recipe) = 330 calories
                                        18 gm protein

## BAKED CHEESE FONDUE

3 eggs, separated
1 can (10 $\frac{1}{2}$ ounces) condensed cream of celery, chicken, or mushroom soup

1 cup shredded sharp Cheddar or process American cheese (4 ounces)
$\frac{1}{4}$ teaspoon dry mustard
2 cups small bread cubes

Heat oven to 325°. Beat egg whites until stiff but not dry. Beat egg yolks until thick and lemon colored. Blend in soup, cheese, and mustard, and stir in bread cubes. Fold into egg whites. Turn into ungreased $1\frac{1}{2}$-quart casserole. Bake 1 hour.

4 to 6 servings      1 serving ($\frac{1}{5}$ recipe) = 225 calories
                                              11 gm protein

*Eggs, Cheese, Pasta, Vegetables*

# BASIC SOUFFLE

1 cup White Sauce (below)
3 eggs, separated

1 cup shredded Cheddar cheese, ground ham, or finely chopped vegetables

Prepare White Sauce. Stir egg yolks and cheese into sauce. Cook over low heat, stirring constantly, until cheese is melted. Remove from heat.

Heat oven to 350°. Beat egg whites until stiff peaks form. Fold egg yolk mixture into egg whites. Turn into greased 1-quart casserole. Bake 20 minutes or until set. Serve immediately.

4 servings   ¼ cheese or meat soufflé = 305 calories
                                            14 gm protein
              ¼ vegetable soufflé = 210 calories
                                            9 gm protein

» *White Sauce:* Melt 3 tablespoons margarine or butter in saucepan over low heat. Blend in 3 tablespoons flour. Cook over low heat, stirring constantly, until mixture is smooth and bubbly. Remove from heat. Stir in 1 cup milk. Heat to boiling, stirring constantly. Boil and stir 1 minute. Remove from heat.

1 cup.

NOTE: This is a standard White Sauce for soufflés.

# CHICKEN PUFF

*Soft and easy to swallow.*

1½ cups chicken broth
¼ cup uncooked cream of rice cereal
2 tablespoons margarine or butter
1 teaspoon oregano leaves, crushed

¼ teaspoon salt
¼ teaspoon pepper sauce
3 eggs, separated
1 cup diced cooked chicken

Heat oven to 325°. Heat chicken broth to boiling in saucepan. Sprinkle cereal on broth; cook, stirring constantly, 1 minute. Remove from heat and let stand 4 minutes. Stir in margarine, salt, oregano, and pepper sauce.

Beat egg whites until stiff but not dry. Beat egg yolks until thick and lemon colored; gradually mix in warm cereal mixture and chicken. Carefully fold in egg whites.

Pour into ungreased 4-cup soufflé dish or 1-quart casserole. Bake until puffed and golden brown, about 45 minutes. Serve immediately.

4 servings     1 serving ($\frac{1}{4}$ soufflé) = 225 calories
                                              17 gm protein

NOTE: Nice served with Creole Sauce (page 204)

## CHEESE RAREBIT

2 cups shredded Cheddar cheese (8 ounces)
$\frac{1}{2}$ cup beer
1 tablespoon margarine or butter
$\frac{1}{4}$ teaspoon dry mustard
$\frac{1}{4}$ teaspoon paprika
1 egg
Toast triangles

Heat cheese, beer, margarine, mustard, and paprika in top of double boiler over hot water, stirring constantly, until cheese is melted. Beat egg slightly; beat into cheese mixture and cook over low heat until thickened, stirring frequently. Serve over toast.

4 servings     1 serving ($\frac{1}{4}$ recipe) = 285 calories
                                              16 gm protein

## CHICKEN QUICHE

*Bland and easy to swallow.*

Pastry for 9-inch one-crust pie (page 228)
1 cup shredded Swiss cheese (4 ounces)
2 tablespoons flour
1 tablespoon instant chicken-flavored bouillon
2 cups cubed cooked chicken
$\frac{1}{4}$ cup chopped onion
2 tablespoons chopped green pepper
2 tablespoons chopped pimiento
3 eggs
1 cup milk

Heat oven to 425°. Prepare pastry. Bake shell 8 minutes, then remove from oven. Reduce oven temperature to 350°. Toss cheese, flour, and bouillon in bowl. Stir in chicken, onion, green pepper, and pimiento. Beat eggs and milk until blended. Mix into cheese-chicken mixture. Pour into pastry shell. Bake 40 to 45 minutes or until set. Let stand 10 minutes before serving.

6 servings     $\frac{1}{6}$ quiche = 290 calories
                              26 gm protein

# QUICHE LORRAINE

Pastry for 9-inch one-crust pie (page 228)
2 cups shredded Swiss cheese (8 ounces)
2 tablespoons flour
4 eggs
1½ cups milk
½ teaspoon salt
Dash cayenne pepper
½ pound bacon, crisply fried and crumbled
Bacon curls (below)
Parsley sprigs

Heat oven to 350°. Prepare pastry. Toss cheese and flour in bowl. Beat eggs, milk, salt, and cayenne pepper. Pour over cheese mixture and stir in crumbled bacon. Pour into pastry-lined pie pan. Bake 40 to 45 minutes. Garnish with bacon curls and parsley sprigs.

6 servings  ⅙ quiche = 420 calories
22 gm protein

» *Bacon Curls:* Cook 6 slices bacon until almost crisp. Roll each slice around tines of fork to make curl; continue to cook until crisp. Drain.

# CREOLE SAUCE OMELET ROLLS

1 tablespoon margarine
1 medium onion, chopped
1 small green pepper, chopped
1 large tomato, peeled and diced
¼ teaspoon paprika
2 teaspoons oregano
Salt and pepper to taste
3 omelet rolls

Prepare 3 omelet rolls, mixing and cooking one at a time as directed on page 154; keep rolls warm on ungreased baking sheet in 275° oven while preparing sauce.

Melt margarine in small saucepan. Cook and stir onion in margarine until tender. Stir in green pepper, tomato, paprika and oregano; season with salt and pepper. Reduce heat; simmer until green pepper is tender, about 10 minutes. Serve ⅓ cup sauce on each omelet roll.

3 servings  1 omelet roll with sauce = 155 calories
8 gm protein

# MUSHROOM OMELET

½ pound fresh mushrooms, sliced
½ cup thinly sliced onion
¼ cup finely chopped green pepper
2 tablespoons vegetable oil
4 eggs
Salt and pepper to taste

Cook and stir mushrooms, onion, and green pepper in oil until onion is tender, 3 to 4 minutes. Mix eggs, salt, and pepper with fork until whites and yolks are just blended. Pour mixture on vegetables in skillet. Slide skillet back and forth rapidly over heat. At the same time, stir quickly with fork to spread egg mixture continuously over bottom of skillet as it thickens. Let stand over heat a few seconds to brown bottom of omelet lightly; do not overcook. (Omelet will continue to cook after folding.)

Tilt skillet; run fork under edge of omelet, then jerk pan sharply to loosen eggs from bottom of skillet. Fold $\frac{1}{3}$ portion of omelet nearest to you just to center. Allow for portion of omelet to slide up side of skillet. Fold opposite $\frac{1}{3}$ portion to center. Turn omelet onto warm plate.

4 servings     1 serving ($\frac{1}{4}$ omelet) = 170 calories
                                              8 gm protein

## OMELET AUX FINES HERBES

3 eggs
2 tablespoons snipped parsley
1 teaspoon snipped fresh or $\frac{1}{2}$ teaspoon dried tarragon leaves
$\frac{1}{2}$ teaspoon snipped fresh or $\frac{1}{4}$ teaspoon dried thyme leaves

$\frac{1}{8}$ teaspoon pepper
2 teaspoons chopped shallots or scallions
1 tablespoon margarine or butter
Salt and pepper to taste

Beat eggs with fork until whites and yolks are just blended. Stir in parsley, tarragon, thyme, pepper, and shallots/scallions. Heat margarine in 8-inch skillet or omelet pan over medium-high heat. As margarine melts, tilt skillet in all directions to coat sides thoroughly. When margarine begins to brown, skillet is hot enough to use.

Quickly pour egg mixture all at once into skillet. With left hand, start sliding skillet back and forth rapidly over heat. At the same time, stir quickly with fork to spread eggs continuously over bottom of skillet as they thicken. Let stand over heat a few seconds to brown bottom of omelet lightly; do not overcook. (Omelet will continue to cook after folding.)

Tilt skillet; run fork under edge of omelet, then jerk skillet sharply to loosen eggs from bottom of skillet. Fold $\frac{1}{3}$ portion of omelet nearest to you just to center. Allow for portion of omelet to slide up side of skillet. Fold opposite $\frac{1}{3}$ portion to center. Turn omelet onto warm plate.

3 servings     1 serving ($\frac{1}{3}$ omelet) = 120 calories
                                              7 gm protein

# OMELET ROLL

1 egg                                        Salt and pepper to taste
1 tablespoon cream or milk

For each roll, beat egg and cream or milk, and salt and pepper to taste with rotary beater.

Melt 2 teaspoons margarine or butter in 10-inch skillet; rotate pan to coat bottom with margarine. Pour egg mixture into skillet; slowly rotate pan to spread mixture into thin circle. Cook over medium heat about 2 minutes. Loosen edge; roll up, using small spatula and fork. Season with salt and pepper.

1 serving        1 roll = 135 calories
                          7 gm protein

### VARIATION

» *Herb Omelet Roll:* Just before rolling egg, sprinkle basil, chervil, thyme, or marjoram leaves and snipped chives on top.

NOTE: When preparing more than one, keep Omelet Roll warm on ungreased baking sheet in 275° oven.

# MUSHROOM-SHRIMP SAUCE WITH OMELET ROLLS

1 tablespoon shrimp spice                    1 teaspoon chopped onion
1½ quarts water (6 cups)                     ¼ cup chopped celery
20 frozen cleaned cooked shrimp (¼           ½ cup sliced fresh mushrooms
  pound, small)                              1 tablespoon lemon juice
½ cup whipping cream                         Salt and pepper to taste
½ cup water                                  4 omelet rolls
1 tablespoon flour

Tie shrimp spice in cheesecloth. Heat 1½ quarts water and shrimp spice to boiling in large saucepan; boil 15 minutes. Add frozen shrimp; heat to boiling and remove from heat. Let shrimp remain in water 5 minutes. Drain; cut up shrimp.

Prepare 4 omelet rolls, mixing and cooking one at a time as directed above; keep rolls warm on ungreased baking sheet in 275° oven while preparing sauce.

Mix cream, ½ cup water, and the flour in medium saucepan until smooth. Cook over low heat, stirring constantly, until mixture thickens and boils. Boil and stir 1 minute.

Stir in onion, celery, and mushrooms; salt and pepper to taste. Reduce heat; simmer, stirring occasionally, until mushrooms are tender, about 10 minutes. Stir in lemon juice and shrimp. Pour $\frac{1}{3}$ cup sauce on each omelet roll.

4 servings        1 omelet roll = 295 calories
                                12 gm protein

## CALIFORNIA SAUCE OMELET ROLLS

$\frac{3}{4}$ cup dairy sour cream
$\frac{1}{8}$ teaspoon dill weed
1 large tomato, peeled and diced

1 small avocado, diced
Salt and pepper to taste
4 omelet rolls

Prepare 4 omelet rolls, mixing and cooking one at a time as directed on page 154; keep rolls warm on ungreased baking sheet in 275° oven while preparing sauce.

Heat sour cream and dill weed. Stir in tomato and avocado; season with salt and pepper. Heat 1 minute and pour $\frac{1}{3}$ cup sauce on each omelet roll.

4 servings        1 roll = 370 calories
                              10 gm protein

## BAKED EGGS

*Tired of plain eggs? Try this easy recipe.*

2 tablespoons margarine or butter
6 eggs
2 tablespoons shredded Cheddar or process American cheese

2 tablespoons crumbled crisp-fried bacon
2 tablespoons snipped parsley

Heat oven to 350°. Place 1 teaspoon margarine in each of six muffin cups. Break one egg into each cup, and sprinkle each with 1 teaspoon of cheese and one of bacon. Top with 1 teaspoon parsley. Bake 15 to 20 minutes, until eggs are desired consistency.

6 servings        1 serving = 135 calories
                              7 gm protein

NOTE: If spicy eggs are desired, sprinkle eggs with salt, pepper, paprika, and dash of Worcestershire sauce or pepper sauce.

# CHEESY CREAMED EGGS

1 can (10½ ounces) condensed
    Cheddar cheese soup or cream
    of celery soup
⅓ cup light cream (20%) or milk

4 hard-cooked eggs, sliced
2 tablespoons chopped pimiento
4 slices toast
Snipped parsley

Blend soup and cream in saucepan. Stir in eggs and pimiento. Heat, stirring constantly, just to simmering. Reduce heat and simmer 5 minutes, stirring frequently. Add more cream for thinner sauce. Serve on toast and garnish with parsley.

4 servings      1 serving (1 slice toast plus ⅓ cup sauce) = 250 calories
                                                 13 gm protein

# EGGS A LA KING

½ cup water
2 tablespoons flour
1 to 1½ teaspoons onion powder
⅛ teaspoon salt
⅛ teaspoon white pepper
½ cup whipping cream
1 to 2 tablespoons lemon juice

¼ cup chopped fresh mushrooms
2 tablespoons chopped green
    pepper
2 tablespoons chopped pimiento
4 hard-cooked eggs, chopped
2 English muffins, split
2 teaspoons margarine or butter

Mix water, flour, onion powder, salt, and pepper in small saucepan until smooth. Stir in cream. Cook over low heat, stirring constantly, until mixture thickens and boils. Boil and stir 1 minute. Remove from heat; stir in lemon juice, mushrooms, green pepper, pimiento, and eggs.

    Toast muffin halves, and spread with margarine. Heat egg mixture and serve on muffin halves.

2 servings      1 serving (½ recipe) = 540 calories
                                      21 gm protein

# BAKED EGGS WITH CHEESE

1 package (3 ounces) cream cheese, softened
6 eggs
¼ teaspoon crushed basil leaves

¼ cup whipping cream
Salt and pepper
¾ cup shredded Cheddar cheese
Snipped parsley

Heat oven to 350°. Cut cream cheese into 6 pieces; place each in greased custard cup or small baking dish. Break one egg into each cup; top each with 2 teaspoons cream and season with salt and pepper. Sprinkle 2 tablespoons Cheddar cheese in each cup. Place cups in pan of hot water (1 inch deep). Bake 15 to 18 minutes, until eggs are desired consistency. Garnish with parsley.

6 servings      1 serving = 220 calories
                           11 gm protein


# OVEN SOUFFLE

*Do the preparation the night before for an easy family breakfast.*

8 slices bread
Margarine or butter, softened
6 eggs
3 cups milk
½ teaspoon salt

¼ teaspoon pepper
Dash paprika
1½ teaspoons Worcestershire sauce
2 cups shredded sharp Cheddar cheese (approximately ½ pound)

Remove crusts from bread slices; spread slices on both sides with margarine and place side by side in baking dish 11½ x 7½ x 1½ inches. Beat eggs, milk, and seasonings; pour over bread. Sprinkle cheese on top, and refrigerate 8 to 12 hours.
   Heat oven to 325°. Bake 40 to 45 minutes, until set.

6 servings      ⅙ soufflé = 380 calories
                           22 gm protein

# COLD CURRIED EGGS

1 tablespoon olive oil
2 teaspoons curry powder
½ cup sherry
1 tablespoon lemon juice
¼ teaspoon white pepper

½ cup mayonnaise
¼ cup chilled whipping cream
6 hard-cooked eggs
1 tablespoon snipped chives

Mix olive oil and curry powder in small saucepan and heat (do not boil). Stir in sherry; heat just to simmer. Simmer until liquid is reduced to half. Remove from heat and cool. Stir curry mixture, pepper, and lemon juice into mayonnaise. Beat cream in chilled bowl until stiff. Fold mayonnaise mixture into cream. Cover and refrigerate at least 3 hours.

Cut eggs lengthwise into halves; remove yolks. Cut whites lengthwise into ⅛-inch slices. Arrange slices in serving dish, and spread with mayonnaise mixture. Press egg yolks through sieve onto top. Sprinkle with chives.

4 servings    1 serving (¼ recipe) = 395 calories
10 gm protein

# EGGS FOO YOUNG

6 eggs
3 tablespoons water
1 tablespoon Worcestershire sauce
⅛ teaspoon salt

1 can (5 ounces) water chestnuts,
drained and coarsely chopped
¼ cup thinly sliced scallions
¼ cup diced green pepper
1 tablespoon margarine or butter

Set oven control at broil or 550°. Beat eggs, water, Worcestershire sauce, and salt with rotary beater. Stir in water chestnuts, scallions, and green pepper.

Melt margarine in large skillet with heat-proof handle. Pour in egg mixture. As mixture begins to set at bottom and side, gently lift cooked portion with spatula so that thin, uncooked portion can flow to bottom. When cooked throughout but still moist, place skillet under broiler. Broil 3 to 4 minutes until light brown. Loosen edge with spatula and slip omelet onto warm plate. Cut into wedges.

4 servings    1 wedge (¼ recipe) = 190 calories
10 gm protein

# BAKED EGGS PROVENÇAL

2 ripe tomatoes
Salt and pepper
Dash garlic salt
2 teaspoons snipped parsley

2 eggs
Margarine or butter
Dash basil
Parmesan cheese

Heat oven to 400°. Cut thin slice from stem end of tomatoes. Remove pulp from tomatoes with curved knife, leaving 1-inch-thick wall. Place tomatoes in greased baking dish. Sprinkle with salt, pepper, garlic salt, and parsley. Bake 10 minutes.

Remove from oven; break an egg into each tomato. Dot with margarine; sprinkle with basil, and bake 20 minutes longer. Sprinkle tops with Parmesan cheese, and bake 10 minutes or until eggs are desired consistency.

2 servings     1 serving = 160 calories
                        8 gm protein


# SHIRRED EGGS WITH MUSHROOMS

$\frac{1}{4}$ cup margarine or butter
2 cups finely chopped fresh
   mushrooms
$\frac{1}{2}$ cup finely chopped onion

6 slices bread
6 eggs
$\frac{3}{4}$ cup light cream (20%)

Heat oven to 350°. Melt 2 tablespoons of the margarine in skillet. Cook and stir mushrooms and onion in margarine over low heat until mushrooms are soft and most of the liquid is absorbed.

Grease six 10-ounce custard cups. Trim crusts from bread slices; toast bread. Spread both sides of toast slices with remaining margarine. Gently place 1 slice toast in each custard cup. Divide mushroom-onion mixture, plus any liquid, among custard cups. Break 1 egg into each cup; sprinkle 2 tablespoons cream on egg. Bake uncovered 20 minutes.

6 servings     1 serving (1 custard cup) = 270 calories
                                    10 gm protein

*Eggs, Cheese, Pasta, Vegetables*

# EGGS BEARNAISE

*As savory dish that makes a special occasion out of any breakfast, lunch, or dinner.*

Béarnaise Sauce (below or use 1
    cup prepared sauce)
6 whole-wheat English muffins,
    split

12 slices Canadian bacon
12 eggs
Paprika
Black Olive slices

Prepare Béarnaise Sauce. Keep warm by placing blender container in pan of warm water. (You can purchase prepared Béarnaise Sauce in the specialty section of the supermarket.) Heat oven to 350°. Arrange muffin halves on baking sheet; bake 1 minute. Top each half with bacon slice. Bake until bacon is warm and edges of muffin halves are brown. Poach eggs. Top each muffin half with an egg. Spoon Béarnaise Sauce over each serving. Garnish with paprika and olive slices.

6 servings     1 serving (1 muffin, 2 eggs) = 495 calories
                                30 gm protein

» *Béarnaise Sauce*

3 egg yolks
2 teaspoons tarragon vinegar
$\frac{1}{4}$ teaspoon onion salt

$\frac{1}{4}$ teaspoon tarragon leaves
$\frac{1}{2}$ cup margarine or butter, melted

Blend egg yolks, vinegar, salt, and tarragon leaves in blender on high speed until smooth, about 2 seconds. Drizzle hot margarine slowly into egg mixture while blending at high speed. To make tarragon vinegar, fill a jar with fresh tarragon leaves and cover with white vinegar. After 24 hours, strain vinegar and cork bottle.

2 cups = 990 calories
          10 gm protein


# BOB'S FAVORITE NOODLE CASSEROLE

*Wonderful as a side dish or as a meatless meal.*

$1\frac{1}{2}$ cups cottage cheese
$1\frac{1}{2}$ cups dairy sour cream
1 clove garlic, crushed
1 small onion, minced
1 tablespoon Worcestershire sauce
Dash pepper sauce
2 teaspoons salt

1 tablespoon plus $1\frac{1}{2}$ teaspoons
    horseradish (optional)
$\frac{1}{4}$ pound sliced bacon
1 package (8 ounces) very fine egg
    noodles or vermicelli
$\frac{1}{2}$ cup grated Parmesan cheese
Parsley

Heat oven to 350°. Mix cottage cheese, sour cream, garlic, onion, Worcestershire sauce, pepper sauce, salt, and horseradish in large bowl. Fry bacon until crisp. Drain and crumble into bowl. Cook noodles as directed on package. Turn noodles into bowl with cottage cheese mixture and toss until noodles are well coated. Turn into greased 2-quart casserole. Cover and bake 30 to 40 minutes, until hot. Remove cover; sprinkle $\frac{1}{4}$ cup of the Parmesan cheese on top.

Set oven control at broil or 550°. Place casserole about 6 inches from heat, and broil until top is golden. Garnish casserole with parsley. Serve with remaining Parmesan cheese in small bowl and with small bowl of dairy sour cream, if desired.

6 servings        1 serving ($\frac{1}{6}$ recipe) = 395 calories
                                    18 gm protein

## FETTUCINI CARBONARA

1 package (12 ounces) fettucini or
   spaghetti
$\frac{1}{4}$ pound sliced bacon
$\frac{1}{4}$ cup margarine or butter, softened

$\frac{1}{2}$ cup whipping cream
$\frac{1}{2}$ cup grated Parmesan cheese
2 eggs slightly beaten
2 tablespoons snipped parsley

Cook fettucini as directed on package. Fry bacon until crisp; drain and crumble into serving bowl. Turn hot fettucini into bowl; add remaining ingredients and toss until fettucini is coated. Serve warm.

6 servings        1 serving ($\frac{1}{6}$ recipe) = 435 calories
                                    18 gm protein

## HAM 'N' CHEESE PIE

*A soft, easy-to-eat main dish.*

8-inch baked pie shell
2 eggs
1 jar ($3\frac{1}{2}$ ounces) junior baby ham
1 can (6 ounces) evaporated milk ($\frac{2}{3}$
   cup)

1 cup shredded Cheddar cheese (4
   ounces)
1 tablespoon instant minced onion

Bake pie shell. Reduce oven temperature to 325°. Beat eggs; stir in remaining ingredients. Pour into pie shell. Bake 30 to 40 minutes or until set.

4 or 5 servings       1 serving ($\frac{1}{5}$ pie) = 240 calories
                                    15 gm protein

*Eggs, Cheese, Pasta, Vegetables*

# HAM AND EGG EN CROUTE

1 package (17½ ounces) frozen puff pastry
1 pound sliced cooked ham, cut into julienne strips
8 eggs
1 package (8 ounces) herbed cheese spread, cut into ¼-inch pieces
1 egg
1 teaspoon water

Thaw pastry 20 minutes. Unfold and cut each sheet into 4 squares. Cut ½-inch hole in center of each square.

Line eight 5-ounce custard cups with half of the ham strips. Break an egg into each cup and top with pieces of cheese spread and remaining ham strips. Top each with a pastry square, pressing pastry edges tightly into cup. Beat one egg slightly with water; brush on tops of pastry. Cover and refrigerate up to 12 hours.

Heat oven to 425°. Bake 15 minutes for soft-cooked yolk; 20 minutes for hard-cooked yolk, until pastry is puffed and golden brown.

8 servings      1 cup = 280 calories
                     21 gm protein

# BEST-EVER SPINACH

2 packages (10 ounces each) frozen chopped spinach
1 package (8 ounces) cream cheese, softened
¼ cup margarine or butter, softened
½ teaspoon celery salt
½ teaspoon garlic salt
Dash pepper sauce
¼ teaspoon salt
Dash pepper
1 can (3 ounces) French fried onions
½ cup bread crumbs
2 tablespoons margarine or butter, melted

Heat oven to 350°. Cook spinach as directed on package. Turn into 1-quart casserole. Mix cream cheese, ½ cup margarine, and the seasoning until smooth; spoon onto spinach. Spread onions over top. Mix bread crumbs and 2 tablespoons margarine; sprinkle over onions. Bake 15 to 20 minutes, until very hot.

8 servings      1 serving (⅛ recipe) = 280 calories
                     5 gm protein

# HAM AND MACARONI BAKE

*A bit more work, but loaded with calories.*

1 package (8 ounces) elbow
    macaroni
2 tablespoons brown sugar
2 cups cubed cooked ham
2 cups thinly sliced apple (2
    medium)
¼ cup margarine
¼ cup whole-wheat flour
2 tablespoons prepared mustard

½ teaspoon salt
Dash pepper
2 cups milk
1 cup shredded Cheddar Cheese (4
    ounces)
3 tablespoons margarine or butter
1 cup soft bread crumbs (about 1
    slice)

Cook macaroni as directed on package. Turn into 2-quart casserole. Stir in sugar, ham, and apple.

Heat oven to 350°. Melt ¼ cup margarine in saucepan. Stir in whole-wheat flour, mustard, salt, and pepper. Cook over low heat, stirring until mixture is bubbly. Remove from heat. Stir in milk. Heat to boiling, stirring constantly. Boil and stir 1 minute. Stir in cheese until melted. Pour over macaroni mixture in casserole and mix. Melt 3 tablespoons margarine; pour over bread crumbs and sprinkle crumbs on casserole. Bake 30 to 35 minutes, until hot and bubbly.

8 servings      1 serving (⅛ recipe) = 515 calories
                              19 gm protein

# EASY HAM AND MACARONI BAKE

1 package (7¼ ounces) macaroni and
    cheese dinner
2 cups cubed cooked ham
2 cups thinly sliced apple

¾ cup soft bread crumbs
1 cup shredded Cheddar cheese (4
    ounces)
2 tablespoons wheat germ

Heat oven to 350°. Cook macaroni and cheese dinner as directed on package. Stir in ham and apple. Turn into 2-quart casserole. Mix bread crumbs, cheese, and wheat germ; sprinkle over top of casserole. Bake 20 minutes.

4 to 6 servings      1 serving (⅙ recipe) = 490 calories
                              25 gm protein

# CRISSCROSS POTATOES

*Spruce up your baked potato with extra protein.*

1 large baking potato
2 tablespoons margarine or butter,
   melted

Freshly ground pepper
$\frac{1}{4}$ cup grated Cheddar cheese
Paprika

Heat oven to 400°. Cut unpared potato lengthwise in half. Make diagonal cuts about $\frac{1}{8}$ inch deep on cut surfaces of potato, forming crisscross pattern. Brush with margarine, and season with pepper. Place in small shallow baking pan. Bake uncovered 40 minutes. Sprinkle with cheese and paprika and bake 10 minutes longer.

2 servings     1 serving ($\frac{1}{2}$ potato) = 230 calories
                                    6 gm protein

# CHEESE NOODLE CASSEROLE

*A smooth side dish with meat or poultry.*

3 eggs
1 cup cooked noodles, approximately 2 ounces
1 cup small bread cubes
1 tablespoon snipped parsley
1 tablespoon chopped pimiento

1 teaspoon chopped onion
$\frac{1}{2}$ cup margarine or butter, melted
$\frac{1}{2}$ cup shredded process American
   or Cheddar cheese
1 cup light cream (20%) or milk

Heat oven to 300°. Beat eggs thoroughly in medium bowl. Stir in remaining ingredients. Turn into ungreased $1\frac{1}{2}$-quart casserole. Place casserole in pan of hot water (1 inch deep). Bake 1 hour.

6 to 8 servings     1 serving (about $\frac{3}{4}$ cup) = 290 calories
                                    7 gm protein

# SPINACH SUPREME

*Not all vegetables are low calorie.*

2 packages (10 ounces each) frozen chopped spinach
$\frac{1}{2}$ cup margarine or butter (1 stick)
1 package (8 ounces) cream cheese, softened

$\frac{1}{2}$ cup bread crumbs
$\frac{3}{4}$ teaspoon sage
Dash freshly ground pepper

Heat oven to 350°. Cook spinach as directed on package. Mix half the margarine and the cream cheese until smooth. Stir in hot spinach. Turn into ungreased 1$\frac{1}{2}$-quart casserole.

Melt remaining margarine; stir in bread crumbs, sage, and pepper and sprinkle on casserole. Bake 20 to 30 minutes.

6 servings        1 serving (a generous $\frac{1}{2}$ cup) = 310 calories
6 gm protein

# 14

## MEAT AND POULTRY

CHERRY SAUCE · TARRAGON VEAL · VEAL OR CHICKEN
PICCATA · VEAL CUTLET PARMESAN · BEEF 'N' BEER
CASSEROLE · CHILI CON CARNE · SPICY JALAPENO MEAT
LOAF · STEAK TERIYAKI · MANICOTTI · STEAK AU POIVRE ·
BEEF PATTIES IN WINE SAUCE · LAZY DAY POT ROAST ·
FRUIT KEBAB GARNISH · SHISH KEBABS · HAMBURGER
STROGANOFF · SPEEDY STROGANOFF · SAUCY MEATBALLS ·
BURGERS BEARNAISE · CHILI · CHILIBURGER · KATHERINE'S
COTTAGE CHEESE MEAT LOAF · POLYNESIAN HASH ·
MARINATED LEMON CHICKEN · BROILED CHICKEN ITALIANO ·
SWEET-AND-SOUR CHICKEN OR PORK · LEMON SESAME
CHICKEN · TASTY BUTTER · CURRIED ORANGE CHCIKEN ·
SPICY CHICKEN BREASTS · CHICKEN-RICE CASSEROLE ·
INSTANT CHICKEN DIVAN · SUMMER GARDEN CHICKEN ·
EFFORTLESS CHICKEN IN WINE · WESTERN CHICKEN · COLD
CURRIED CHICKEN · COLD CHINESE CHICKEN · COMPANY
CHICKEN CASSEROLE · CREAMED CHICKEN · CHICKEN A LA
KING · TURKEY STROGANOFF · CHEESE TURKEY CASSEROLE ·
CHICKEN OR TURKEY TETRAZZINI

# CHERRY SAUCE

½ cup currant jelly
1 can (16 ounces) pitted red tart
   cherries, drained (reserve
   liquid)

½ cup brown sugar (packed)
¼ teaspoon cloves
¼ teaspoon cinnamon
Grated peel and juice of ½ lemon

Melt jelly in small saucepan over low heat, stirring constantly. Stir in cherries, sugar, cloves, cinnamon, and peel and juice of lemon. Heat, stirring occasionally. Stir in reserved liquid, small amount at a time, until sauce is desired consistency. Serve hot or cold on roast meats.

3 cups     ¼ cup = 90 calories
                     0 protein


# TARRAGON VEAL

*A piquant taste is added to an ordinarily bland dish.*

1½ pounds cooked veal, sliced
¼ cup margarine or butter
¼ cup all-purpose flour
¼ teaspoon pepper

¼ teaspoon paprika
1¼ cups water
¾ cup white wine
1 teaspoon tarragon leaves

Heat oven to 325°. Arrange meat in ungreased baking dish, 11¾ x 7½ x 1½ inches. Melt margarine in saucepan over low heat; stir in flour, pepper, and paprika. Cook over low heat, stirring until mixture is smooth and bubbly. Remove from heat. Stir in water and wine. Heat to boiling, stirring constantly. Sprinkle tarragon on meat and pour sauce on top. Cover and bake until hot and bubbly, about 30 minutes.

8 servings.    1 serving (approximately 3 ounces) = 205 calories
                                         19 gm protein

# VEAL OR CHICKEN PICCATA

6 thin slices boneless veal steak
(about 1½ pounds) or 3 chicken
breasts, split, boned, skinned,
and pounded thin; or 6 chicken
cutlets
1 teaspoon salt
¼ cup margarine

⅓ cup white wine, vermouth, or
chicken broth
6 thin lemon slices
1 teaspoon dried tarragon leaves
3 cups hot cooked rice
2 tablespoons snipped parsley

Season meat with salt. Melt margarine in large skillet; brown meat
on both sides. Pour wine over meat; arrange lemon slices on meat
and sprinkle with tarragon leaves. Heat to boiling. Reduce heat,
cover, and simmer 2 to 3 minutes or until meat is tender. Serve over
rice and sprinkle parsley on top.

6 servings     1 serving (approximately 3½ ounces) = 370 calories
27 gm protein

# VEAL CUTLET PARMESAN

4 boneless veal cutlets (about 4
ounces each) or 1 pound veal
steak, ½ inch thick
1 cup bread crumbs
2 tablespoons grated Parmesan
cheese

2 eggs
1 teaspoon salt
Dash pepper
3 tablespoons olive oil
1 can (8 ounces) tomato sauce
4 slices mozzarella cheese

Heat oven to 350°. If using veal steak, cut into 4 pieces. Mix bread
crumbs and Parmesan cheese. Beat eggs, salt, and pepper until
blended. Heat oil in large skillet. Dip meat into egg mixture, then
into bread crumb mixture. Brown in skillet on both sides, about 8
minutes. Place in baking pan 9 x 9 x 2 inches; top with tomato sauce
and slices of mozzarella. Bake 10 to 15 minutes or until meat is
tender.

4 servings     1 serving = 540 calories
39 gm protein

# BEEF 'N' BEER CASSEROLE

*This can be made several days before serving.*

3 tablespoons olive oil
3 pounds beef stew meat
½ teaspoon salt
Freshly ground pepper
¼ cup plus 2 tablespoons margarine
   or butter
1 cup thinly sliced mushrooms or 1

can (6 ounces) sliced mushrooms, drained
6 medium onions, thinly sliced
3 tablespoons flour
12 ounces beer
1 teaspoon black pepper
½ to 1 teaspoon pepper sauce

Heat oil in large skillet. Brown meat in oil over medium-high heat. Season with salt and pepper. Remove meat to Dutch oven.

Melt margarine in same skillet. Add mushrooms and onions, and sprinkle with flour. Cook and stir mushrooms and onions in margarine until onions are tender. Turn into Dutch oven; add beer.

Simmer uncovered over low heat, stirring occasionally, until meat is tender, about 2 hours. Stir in 1 teaspoon pepper and the pepper sauce. Cool; cover tightly and refrigerate 8 hours.

To serve, heat covered over medium heat until meat mixture simmers.

8 servings    1 serving (4 to 5 ounces beef) = 450 calories
40 gm protein

NOTE: This dish can be prepared up to 5 days in advance. The flavor improves with time.

# CHILI CON CARNE

1 pound ground lean beef
1 can (28 ounces) whole tomatoes
   in thick tomato purée
2 medium onions, chopped (about
   1 cup)
1 clove garlic, crushed
1 tablespoon chili powder

1 teaspoon salt
1 teaspoon sugar
1 teaspoon crushed oregano leaves
1 teaspoon Worcestershire sauce
1 can (20 ounces) red kidney beans,
   drained

Cook and stir meat in large saucepan until brown. Drain off fat and stir in remaining ingredients, breaking up tomatoes with fork or spoon. Heat to boiling. Reduce heat to simmer, cover, and cook 3 hours, stirring occasionally.

6 servings    1 serving (approximately 1 cup) = 250 calories
25 gm protein

# SPICY JALAPEÑO MEAT LOAF

2 eggs
1 can (7½ ounces) tomatoes with
   jalapeños (about ⅔ cup)
2 tablespoons chili powder
2 teaspoons cumin

1 teaspoon salt
1 cup fresh bread crumbs (about 1
   slice)
1 pound ground lean beef

Heat oven to 350°. Beat eggs, tomatoes with jalapeños, seasonings, and bread crumbs in bowl; add meat and mix thoroughly with hands. Shape into loaf in pie pan or turn mixture into loaf pan 8 x 4 x 2½ inches. Bake 40 to 45 minutes, until done and brown.

4 servings     1 serving (2 slices) = 335 calories
                               37 gm protein

NOTE: For individual portions, press ¼ of meat mixture into 6-ounce custard cup. Unmold onto sheet of heavy-duty aluminum foil and seal securely. Repeat with remaining mixture, and freeze. To serve, thaw one or two molds at room temperature about 35 minutes. Unwrap and bake on pie pan in 350° oven for 30 to 40 minutes or until done.

# STEAK TERIYAKI

*Taste-tempting as appetizer or entree.*

⅓ cup soy sauce
⅓ cup saki or sherry
3 tablespoons sugar

1 teaspoon ginger
2½ pound beef steak, 2 inches thick

Mix soy sauce, saki, sugar, and ginger. Pour over steak, cover, and marinate at least 4 hours, turning occasionally.

    Set oven control at broil or 550°. Remove steak from marinade, reserving marinade. Broil steak 4 inches from heat, basting occasionally with marinade, about 15 minutes on each side for medium rare, or until desired degree of doneness.

4 eight-ounce servings or
8 four-ounce servings    1 eight-ounce serving = 450 calories
                                     50 gm protein
                    1 four-ounce serving = 225 calories
                                     25 gm protein

# MANICOTTI

1 carton (8 ounces) cottage cheese
or ricotta cheese
1 cup shredded mozzarella cheese
(4 ounces)
$\frac{1}{2}$ teaspoon salt
$\frac{1}{2}$ cup mayonnaise
$\frac{3}{4}$ pound ground lean beef

1 clove garlic, pressed, or $\frac{1}{8}$ teaspoon garlic powder
8 manicotti, cooked and drained
2 cups tomato sauce
$\frac{1}{2}$ teaspoon oregano
$\frac{1}{3}$ cup grated Parmesan cheese

Mix cottage cheese, mozzarella cheese, salt, and mayonnaise in
bowl. Cook and stir meat and garlic in skillet until meat is brown.
Drain off fat. Stir meat into cottage cheese mixture.

Heat oven to 325°. Fill each manicotti with about $\frac{1}{4}$ cup meat-
cheese filling. Arrange in single layer in baking dish $11\frac{1}{2}$ x $7\frac{1}{2}$ x $1\frac{1}{2}$
inches. Sprinkle any remaining filling on filled manicotti. Pour
tomato sauce on manicotti and sprinkle with oregano and Parmesan
cheese. Cover baking dish with aluminum foil. Bake 15 minutes.
Remove foil and bake 10 minutes longer.

4 servings     1 serving (2 manicotti with sauce) = 617 calories
44 gm protein

NOTE: Individual portions can be wrapped in aluminum foil and
frozen. Heat frozen foil-wrapped portions in 325° oven.

# STEAK AU POIVRE

12-ounce boneless beef steak
$\frac{1}{4}$ teaspoon salt
2 tablespoons peppercorns,
cracked, or coarsely ground
pepper

2 to 3 teaspoons margarine or
butter
2 tablespoons brandy or whiskey

Rub meat with salt and pepper, pressing pepper into meat with
heel of hand. Melt margarine in large skillet. Brown meat in margarine over medium-high heat. Reduce heat; cook meat to desired
doneness. Remove to warm platter. Heat brandy in skillet (do not
boil), stir, and pour over meat.

4 servings     1 serving (3 ounces) = 230 calories
21 gm protein

# BEEF PATTIES IN WINE SAUCE

1 tablespoon margarine or butter
½ medium onion, finely chopped
1 clove garlic, finely chopped
3 tablespoons flour
¾ cup red Burgundy or claret

¼ cup water
Freshly ground pepper
4 beef patties (4 ounces each),
  browned

Melt margarine in skillet; cook and stir onion and garlic in margarine 5 minutes. Stir in flour; cook, stirring constantly, until mixture is bubbly. Remove from heat, and stir in wine and water. Heat to boiling, stirring constantly. Reduce heat; simmer uncovered 15 minutes. Season with salt and pepper.

Heat oven to 325°. Place browned beef patties in ungreased baking pan 10 x 6 x 1½ inches. Pour wine sauce on patties. Cover and bake 30 minutes.

4 servings      1 serving (1 patty with sauce) = 295 calories
                                              21 gm protein

# LAZY DAY POT ROAST

*Put it in the oven and forget about dinner for the rest of the day.*

1 tablespoon vegetable oil
2-pound beef round steak, 1 inch
  thick
2 cups water
1 onion, chopped
1 can (8 ounces) tomatoes

1 tablespoon sugar
1 teaspoon allspice
½ teaspoon basil leaves
1 slice lemon
Salt and pepper

Heat oil in large skillet. Brown meat in oil over medium-high heat. Add remaining ingredients. Reduce heat, cover, and simmer until meat is tender, about 3 hours.

8 servings      1 serving (approximately 3½ ounces) = 360 calories
                                              26 gm protein

---

### FRUIT KEBAB GARNISH

Place one pineapple chunk, one cantaloupe ball, one honeydew melon ball, and one strawberry on wooden skewer. Serve as a garnish with meat, poultry, or fish.

---

# SHISH KEBABS

3 ounces lean beef or lamb cubes
1 small onion, quartered
3 cherry tomatoes
3 mushroom caps
$\frac{1}{2}$ green pepper, cut into 1-inch
    pieces

1 ounce catsup
$\frac{1}{2}$ cup white vinegar
1 teaspoon sugar
Salt and pepper to taste
Hot cooked rice

Alternate pieces of meat, onion, tomatoes, mushrooms, and green pepper on skewers. Mix catsup, vinegar, and sugar; season mixture with salt and pepper; and brush on kebabs. Cook on grill or broil in oven to desired degree of doneness. Serve on rice.

1 serving      1 serving = 310 calories
                         24 gm protein

# HAMBURGER STROGANOFF

1 pound ground lean beef
1 tablespoon margarine or butter
1 can (4 ounces) mushroom stems
    and pieces, drained (reserve
    liquid)
2 tablespoons chopped onion
2 tablespoons flour

$1\frac{1}{2}$ cups beef broth
$\frac{1}{2}$ teaspoon salt
Dash pepper
1 tablespoon catsup
$\frac{1}{2}$ cup dairy sour cream
1 package (8 ounces) egg noodles
Snipped parsley

Cook and stir meat, onion, and mushrooms in margarine until meat is brown. Stir in flour; cook about 2 minutes, stirring constantly. Stir in beef broth, reserved mushroom liquid, salt, pepper, and catsup. Heat to boiling, stirring constantly. Reduce heat and simmer 10 minutes, stirring occasionally.

    Cook noodles as directed on package. Blend sour cream into meat mixture; heat 1 minute. Serve over noodles and sprinkle with parsley.

4 servings      1 serving (approximately $\frac{3}{4}$ cup
            sauce with noodles) = 490 calories
                            36 gm protein

NOTE: Use canned beef broth or make broth by dissolving 2 beef bouillon cubes in $1\frac{1}{2}$ cups boiling water.

# SPEEDY STROGANOFF

*You thought the first one was the quickest stroganoff ever? Try this when you really don't want to stay in the kitchen.*

1½ pounds ground round steak
½ cup chopped onion
2 tablespoons margarine or butter
1 can (10½ ounces) condensed cream of mushroom soup

¼ cup water
½ cup dairy sour cream
½ teaspoon paprika
Hot cooked noodles

Cook and stir meat and onion in margarine in skillet until meat is brown. Stir in soup, water, sour cream, and paprika. Heat, stirring constantly, just to simmering. Reduce heat and simmer about 5 minutes, stirring frequently. Serve over noodles cooked according to package directions.

4 servings      1 serving (¼ recipe) = 440 calories
42 gm protein


# SAUCY MEATBALLS

*A flavorful change from the usual.*

1 pound ground lean beef
⅔ cup grated Parmesan cheese
½ cup seasoned bread crumbs
½ cup milk
1 egg
2 tablespoons shortening
1 tablespoon flour

1 can (28 ounces) tomatoes, in chunks
⅓ cup steak sauce
1 tablespoon sugar
½ teaspoon salt
Hot buttered noodles

Mix meat, cheese, bread crumbs, milk, and egg thoroughly. Shape mixture by tablespoonsful into 20 meatballs. Melt shortening in large skillet. Brown meatballs in skillet. Drain fat from skillet, sprinkle flour over meatballs, and stir in tomatoes, steak sauce, sugar, and salt. Heat to simmering, reduce heat, and simmer uncovered 25 minutes or until sauce is desired consistency. Serve meatballs and sauce over noodles.

5 servings      1 serving (4 meatballs with sauce) = 380 calories
32 gm protein

# BURGERS BEARNAISE

2 cups Béarnaise Sauce
1 pound ground round steak
2 tablespoons margarine or butter

4 slices bread
1 tomato, peeled and diced

Prepare Béarnaise Sauce as directed on page 206 or purchase prepared sauce at your supermarket. Shape meat into 4 patties. Set oven control at broil or 550°. Broil patties 3 inches from heat 3 to 4 minutes on each side for rare, 4 to 7 minutes for well done.

Melt margarine in skillet and brown bread on both sides. Place a patty on each bread slice and top with diced tomato and sauce.

4 servings        1 serving = 720 calories
                                 31 gm protein


# CHILI

1½ pounds ground lean beef
2 cups chopped onion
1 medium green pepper, chopped
2 large garlic cloves, minced
1 can (28 ounces) tomatoes, in
   chunks
1 can (8 ounces) tomato sauce

2 cups water
2 tablespoons chili powder
1 tablespoon salt
1 bay leaf
¼ teaspoon pepper sauce
2 cans (15 ounces each) chili beans

Cook and stir meat, onion, green pepper, and garlic until meat is brown. Stir in remaining ingredients except beans. Heat to boiling, stirring occasionally. Reduce heat, cover, and simmer 1½ hours. Stir in beans, and simmer 30 minutes longer. Thin slices of sharp cheese add a high note to each serving.

6 servings        1 serving (⅙ recipe) = 410 calories
                                           35 gm protein


# CHILIBURGER

1 pound lean ground beef
1 tablespoon shortening
1 can (11½ ounces) condensed bean-
   with-bacon soup

½ cup catsup
½ teaspoon chili powder
6 hamburger buns, split and
   toasted

Cook and stir meat in shortening until meat is brown. Stir in soup, catsup, and chili powder. Heat, stirring constantly, to boiling. Reduce heat and simmer 5 minutes, stirring frequently. (If chili is dry, stir in small amount of water for desired consistency.) Serve on buns.

6 servings     1 serving ($\frac{1}{6}$ recipe on 1 bun) = 390 calories
                                              20 gm protein

## KATHERINE'S COTTAGE CHEESE MEAT LOAF

1 pound ground lean beef
1 cup cottage cheese
1 egg
$\frac{1}{2}$ cup rolled oats
$\frac{1}{4}$ cup catsup

1 tablespoon prepared mustard
2 tablespoons chopped onion
$\frac{3}{4}$ teaspoon salt
$\frac{1}{8}$ teaspoon pepper
$\frac{1}{3}$ cup grated Parmesan cheese

Heat oven to 350°. Mix meat, cottage cheese, eggs, rolled oats, catsup, mustard, onion, and seasonings. Press mixture loosely in baking pan 8 x 8 x 2 inches. Bake 20 minutes. Remove from oven, sprinkle Parmesan cheese on top, and bake 10 minutes longer. Let stand 5 minutes before serving.

4 or 5 servings     1 serving (approximately
                    $1\frac{1}{4}$ inch slice) = 290 calories
                                          35 gm protein

## POLYNESIAN HASH

2 tablespoons pineapple juice
$\frac{1}{8}$ teaspoon dry mustard
1 cup finely chopped cooked pork
$\frac{1}{2}$ cup finely chopped cooked sweet
   potato

1 fresh or canned pineapple slice,
   quartered
$1\frac{1}{2}$ teaspoons brown sugar
$1\frac{1}{2}$ teaspoons margarine or butter

Heat oven to 350°. Mix pineapple juice and mustard in mixing bowl. Stir in meat and sweet potato. Pour into greased 1-quart casserole. Top with pineapple, sprinkle with brown sugar, and dot with margarine. Bake uncovered 30 minutes.

2 servings     1 serving ($\frac{1}{2}$ recipe) = 365 calories
                                       17 gm protein

*Meat and Poultry*

# MARINATED LEMON CHICKEN

*Do the major preparation ahead.*

2¼ to 3-pound broiler-fryer, cut up
¼ cup soy sauce
2 tablespoons white wine
2 tablespoons lemon juice

½ teaspoon pepper sauce
2 green onions, finely chopped
1 clove garlic, crushed

Mix seasoning ingredients in a plastic bag and add chicken parts. Tie bag securely, and refrigerate 6 to 8 hours, turning bag occasionally.

Set oven control at broil or 550°. Place chicken parts on rack in broiler pan, reserving marinade. Broil 8 to 10 inches from heat for 15 minutes. Turn chicken, baste with marinade, and broil 15 minutes longer. (This chicken can also be grilled.)

4 to 6 servings      1 serving (approximately 4½ ounces) = 315 calories
35 gm protein


# BROILED CHICKEN ITALIANO

2 to 2½-pound broiler-fryer, cut into
   quarters

½ cup Italian dressing

Set oven control at broil or 550°. Arrange chicken on rack in broiler pan. Brush with dressing. Broil 4 to 6 inches from heat 45 minutes, basting occasionally, until chicken is tender and brown.

4 servings      1 serving (one quarter chicken) = 350 calories
35 gm protein


# SWEET-AND-SOUR CHICKEN OR PORK

1 pound boneless chicken or pork,
   cut into 1-inch cubes
2 tablespoons vegetable oil
1 can (20 ounces) pineapple chunks
   in unsweetened juice
½ cup corn syrup
¼ cup cider vinegar
2 tablespoons catsup

2 tablespoons soy sauce
1 clove garlic, crushed
1 small green pepper, cut into 1-
   inch squares
2 tablespoons cornstarch
2 tablespoons water
Hot cooked rice or Chinese
   noodles

Brown meat in oil in large skillet over medium heat. Add pineapple chunks (with juice), corn syrup, vinegar, catsup, soy sauce, and garlic. Heat to boiling, stirring occasionally. Reduce heat and simmer 10 minutes until meat is tender, stirring occasionally. Stir in green pepper. Mix cornstarch and water; stir into meat mixture. Heat to boiling, stirring constantly. Boil and stir 1 minute. Serve over rice.

4 servings     1 serving (3 ounces chicken) = 610 calories
                                              23 gm protein

## LEMON SESAME CHICKEN

$2\frac{1}{2}$-pound broiler-fryer chicken, cut    $\frac{1}{4}$ teaspoon rosemary leaves
    up                                          $\frac{1}{4}$ teaspoon thyme
$\frac{1}{4}$ cup lemon juice                    $\frac{1}{4}$ teaspoon marjoram
2 tablespoons vegetable oil                      $\frac{1}{4}$ teaspoon sesame seed
$\frac{1}{2}$ teaspoon dry mustard               $\frac{1}{4}$ teaspoon pepper

Heat oven to 300°. Arrange chicken in lightly greased broiler pan. Mix remaining ingredients; brush part of mixture on chicken. Bake uncovered, brushing frequently with remaining mixture, 1 hour.

Increase oven temperature to 500°. Bake chicken 15 minutes longer.

6 servings     1 serving (approximately 4 ounces) = 290 calories
                                                   31 gm protein

---

### TASTY BUTTER

Guaranteed to boost your appetite, and calories too.

1 stick margarine or butter            1 tablespoon snipped parsley
1 teaspoon lemon juice                 $\frac{1}{4}$ teaspoon tarragon leaves
$\frac{1}{4}$ teaspoon prepared hot mustard    1 tablespoon snipped chives
    (English style)                    Dash freshly ground pepper

Soften margarine with fork. Blend in remaining ingredients. Shape margarine mixture into stick and place in freezer or refrigerate until firm. (Do not freeze.) Cut into squares or slices to give a dash of flavor to vegetables or meat.

6 to 8 servings     1 tablespoon = 100 calories
                                   0 protein

---

# CURRIED ORANGE CHICKEN

2-pound broiler-fryer chicken, cut
  up
½ teaspoon curry powder
⅓ cup orange juice
2 tablespoons honey

2 teaspoons dry mustard
2 teaspoons cornstarch
1 tablespoon water
½ orange, pared and sectioned

Heat oven to 375°. Rub chicken pieces with curry powder. Place skin-side down in ungreased baking dish, 10 x 6 x 1½ inches. Heat orange juice, honey, and mustard in small saucepan, just to simmering, stirring constantly. Pour on chicken. Bake uncovered 30 minutes. Turn chicken, and bake until tender, about 20 minutes.

Remove chicken to serving platter; keep warm. Mix cornstarch and water in small saucepan; stir in pan juices from chicken. Cook over medium heat, stirring constantly, until mixture thickens and boils. Boil and stir 1 minute. Stir in orange sections and heat. Serve chicken with hot cooked rice and pass the orange sauce.

**4 servings**    1 serving (approximately 4½ ounces) = 335 calories
35 gm protein


# SPICY CHICKEN BREASTS

2 chicken breasts, halved and
  boned
2 tablespoons margarine or butter
2 tablespoons vegetable oil
¼ cup dry white wine or chicken
  broth

2 tablespoons prepared French
  mustard
1 cup dairy sour cream
2 cups hot cooked rice or noodles

Remove skin from chicken. Melt margarine in oil in large skillet. Add chicken and cook over medium heat until brown on all sides. Pour wine over chicken and cook 3 minutes. Mix mustard and ½ cup of the sour cream. Pour over chicken and heat to boiling. Reduce heat, cover, and simmer 20 minutes or until chicken is tender. Stir in remaining sour cream and heat through. Serve with rice.

**4 servings**    1 serving (3 ounces chicken with rice
and sauce) = 520 calories
29 gm protein

# CHICKEN-RICE CASSEROLE

*Peanuts add flavor and calories.*

2½ to 3-pound broiler-fryer, cut up
1 tablespoon salt
½ cup margarine or butter
½ teaspoon salt
¼ teaspoon pepper

1 teaspoon marjoram
1 cup uncooked regular rice
¼ cup chopped salted peanuts
¼ cup raisins
4 cups chicken broth

Place chicken in large bowl; cover with water and add 1 tablespoon salt. Set aside.

Heat oven to 350°. Melt margarine, and stir in ½ teaspoon salt, the pepper, and marjoram. Pour half the margarine mixture into baking pan 13 x 9 x 2 inches. Sprinkle rice, peanuts, and raisins in pan. Heat 3 cups of the chicken broth to boiling; pour into pan and stir ingredients. Cover and bake 30 minutes.

Remove chicken from water and pat dry. Arrange on rice and brush with half the remaining margarine mixture. Cover and bake 30 minutes longer, brushing with remaining margarine mixture. Increase oven temperature to 425°. Remove cover, pour in remaining chicken broth, and continue baking chicken 30 minutes, until tender and brown.

6 servings      1 serving (⅙ recipe) = 730 calories
43 gm protein

NOTE: Use canned chicken broth or make broth by dissolving 4 chicken flavored bouillon cubes in 4 cups boiling water.


# INSTANT CHICKEN DIVAN

1 package frozen patty shells
1 can (10½ ounces) condensed cream
  of chicken soup

1 can (10½ ounces) condensed cream
  of mushroom soup
1½ cups cut-up cooked chicken
¾ cup chopped cooked broccoli

Bake patty shells as directed on package. Heat soups, stirring constantly, just to simmering. Stir in chicken and broccoli and let simmer until heated through stirring frequently. Serve in patty shells.

4 to 6 servings      1 serving (1 patty shell with
⅕ sauce) = 240 calories
17 gm protein

# SUMMER GARDEN CHICKEN

*Make ahead and bake later.*

1 teaspoon vegetable oil
3 to 4-ounce chicken piece (leg,
   thigh, breast)
1 small potato, pared and quartered
1 small tomato
1 small onion
2 fresh mushrooms

2 slices green pepper
2 tablespoons uncooked instant rice
1 tablespoon lemon juice
$\frac{1}{8}$ teaspoon paprika
$\frac{1}{8}$ teaspoon dry mustard
Salt and pepper to taste

Heat oven to 450°. Heat oil in small skillet. Brown chicken in oil over medium-high heat. Place browned chicken on piece of double thickness aluminum foil, cover with vegetables, and sprinkle with rice. Mix remaining ingredients, and pour over chicken and vegetables. Fold foil together and seal securely. (At this point, chicken can be refrigerated 3 to 4 hours.)

    Place package in shallow baking pan. Bake, turning every 20 minutes, until chicken and vegetables are tender, about 1 hour and 15 minutes. (Increase baking time by 15 minutes if package has been refrigerated.)

1 serving      1 package = 410 calories
                              32 gm protein


# EFFORTLESS CHICKEN IN WINE

Four 3 to 4-ounce chicken pieces
   (leg, thigh, breast)
Vegetable oil
Salt and pepper to taste

Paprika
1 can condensed cream of mushroom soup, undiluted
$\frac{1}{2}$ cup cooking sherry

Set oven control at broil or 550°. Place chicken pieces on ungreased baking sheet. Brush with oil and season with salt, pepper, and paprika. Broil 7 to 9 inches from heat until brown.

    Heat oven to 350°. Place chicken in ungreased baking dish 8 x 8 x 2 inches. Mix soup and sherry and pour over chicken. Cover and bake until tender, about 1 hour. Serve with rice.

4 servings      1 serving (1 piece) = 260 calories
                                       26 gm protein

# WESTERN CHICKEN

1 package (4 ounces) sliced dried
    beef
4 chicken breasts, skinned, boned,
    and cut into halves
8 bacon slices

1 can (10½ ounces) condensed cream
    of chicken soup
1 carton (4 ounces) dairy sour
    cream

Soak dried beef slices in warm water 15 minutes. Heat oven to 300°. Drain dried beef thoroughly. Line baking dish, 13 x 9 x 2 inches, with slices. Wrap each breast piece with two bacon slices, and arrange in baking dish. Blend soup and sour cream; pour over chicken pieces. Bake 2 hours, until tender and golden brown.

8 servings     1 serving (1 breast with sauce) = 280 calories

31 gm protein

# COLD CURRIED CHICKEN

*Prepare in the morning.*

3 chicken breasts, boned and cut
    into halves
1 tablespoon margarine or butter
1 tablespoon flour
⅛ teaspoon salt

⅛ teaspoon pepper
1 cup chicken broth
1 cup light cream (20%)
1 egg yolk
½ tablespoon curry powder

Heat oven to 350°. Place chicken breasts in a small baking dish, and bake 1 hour or until tender. Cool.

    Melt margarine in saucepan. Stir in flour, salt, and pepper. Cook over low heat, stirring until mixture is smooth and bubbly. Stir in chicken broth and cream. Heat to boiling, stirring constantly. Boil and stir 1 minute. Beat egg yolk and stir in small amount of hot sauce; then stir egg mixture back into saucepan. Heat, stirring constantly, just to boiling. Stir in curry powder. Cool. Pour over chicken and refrigerate at least 4 hours.

6 servings.     1 serving (1 piece) = 250 calories

23 gm protein

NOTE: Use canned broth or make broth by dissolving 2 chicken bouillon cubes in 2 cups boiling water.

# COLD CHINESE CHICKEN

2½ to 3-pound broiler fryer
1 tablespoon salt
2 slices fresh ginger

½ stalk leek or 2 scallions
½ cup Chinese wine or sherry
¼ cup soy sauce

Heat oven to 425°. Rub chicken with salt and put ginger slices and leed in cavity. Place chicken breast-side up in middle of large sheet of heavy-duty aluminum foil. Bring ends of foil up over breast of chicken and overlap 2 inches. Close ends securely and seal by pinching. Place in baking pan. Bake 20 to 30 minutes or until tender. Chicken is done when thickest parts are fork-tender, and drumstick meat feels soft when pressed between fingers. Open foil wrap and cool. Pour wine and soy sauce over chicken and refrigerate 12 hours. Serve cold, sliced.

6 servings        1 serving (about 3½ ounces chicken) = 245 calories
27 gm protein


# COMPANY CHICKEN CASSEROLE

*Lots of texture and tasty too.*

8 whole chicken breasts, cut into
  halves
1 package (6 ounces) chow mein
  noodles
3 cans (10½ ounces each) condensed
  cream of mushroom soup

1 jar (12 ounces) cashew nuts
¾ cup chicken broth
3 cups chopped celery
¾ cup chopped onion

Heat oven to 350°. Place chicken breasts in baking dish 13½ x 9 x 2 inches. Bake 1 hour or until tender. Cool, remove skin and bones, and cut meat into large pieces.

Reserve about ½ cup noodles to sprinkle over casserole. Mix remaining noodles and ingredients. Turn into ungreased 3-quart casserole. Sprinkle reserved noodles over top. Bake 45 minutes or until bubbly.

12 servings        1 serving (1½ breast) = 405 calories
38 gm protein

NOTE: You might want to halve this recipe for family only.

# CREAMED CHICKEN

¼ cup minced onion
½ cup finely chopped celery
2 tablespoons margarine or butter
1 can (10½ ounces) condensed cream
    of chicken soup
½ cup light cream (20%)
⅛ teaspoon sage

2 cans (5 ounces each) boned
    chicken or turkey or 2 cups
    diced cooked chicken or turkey
1 cup peas
4 squares corn bread or 4 slices
    toast
Snipped parsley

Cook and stir onion and celery in margarine until tender. Stir in soup, cream, sage, and chicken. Heat, stirring constantly, just to simmering. Stir in peas. Reduce heat and simmer about 10 minutes. Serve over corn bread squares and sprinkle with parsley.

4 servings     1 serving = 440 calories
                           30 gm protein

# CHICKEN A LA KING

2 tablespoons margarine or butter
4 ounces cut-up cooked chicken
2 tablespoons diced green pepper
½ cup sliced mushrooms
½ cup chicken broth
2 tablespoons flour

½ teaspoon salt
½ cup whipping cream
2 teaspoons lemon juice
2 English muffins, split, or 4 round
    rusks
2 teaspoons margarine or butter

Melt 2 tablespoons margarine in small saucepan. Cook and stir chicken, green pepper, and mushrooms in margarine 5 minutes. Remove from heat. Mix chicken broth, flour, and sage until smooth. Stir flour mixture and whipping cream into saucepan. Cook over low heat, stirring constantly, until mixture thickens and boils. Remove from heat; stir in lemon juice.

    Toast muffin halves; spread 2 teaspoons margarine on halves. Serve hot chicken mixture on muffin halves.

2 servings     1 serving (1 muffin and half the sauce) = 575 calories
                                        26 gm protein

# TURKEY STROGANOFF

*A moist, easy-to-swallow treat.*

$\frac{1}{4}$ cup chopped green pepper
2 tablespoons chopped onion
2 tablespoons margarine or butter
1 can (10$\frac{1}{2}$ ounces) condensed cream
    of mushroom soup
$\frac{1}{2}$ cup dairy sour cream

$\frac{1}{4}$ cup milk
2 cups cooked noodles
1$\frac{1}{2}$ cups diced cooked turkey or
    chicken
$\frac{1}{2}$ teaspoon paprika

Heat oven to 350°. Cook and stir green pepper and onion in margarine until tender. Blend soup, sour cream, and milk in 1$\frac{1}{2}$-quart casserole. Stir in green pepper mixture and remaining ingredients. Bake 35 minutes.

4 servings      1 serving ($\frac{1}{2}$ recipe) = 390 calories
                                             23 gm protein

# CHEESE TURKEY CASSEROLE

1 package (8 ounces) egg noodles
2 cups cut-up cooked turkey or
    chicken
1 can (16 ounces) tomato sauce
1 package (8 ounces) cream cheese,
    softened

1 carton (8 ounces) cottage cheese
$\frac{1}{3}$ cup chopped green onion
1 tablespoon chopped green
    pepper

Cook noodles as directed on package. Heat turkey and tomato sauce to simmering. Reduce heat and simmer 10 minutes. Mix cream cheese, cottage cheese, onion, and green pepper.

Heat oven to 350°. Layer half the noodles in buttered 2-quart casserole, then add the cheese mixture, remaining noodles, and the turkey mixture. Bake 30 minutes.

8 servings      1 serving (about 1 cup) = 310 calories
                                             21 gm protein

# CHICKEN OR TURKEY TETRAZZINI

1 package (8 ounces) spaghetti
1 cup water
2 tablespoons flour
1 cup whipping cream
1 chicken bouillon cube
$\frac{1}{4}$ cup margarine or butter
2 tablespoons red wine vinegar

$\frac{1}{4}$ teaspoon salt
Pepper to taste
2 cups cut-up cooked chicken or
  turkey
$\frac{3}{4}$ cup sliced mushrooms
2 tablespoons grated Parmesan
  cheese

Heat oven to 350°. Cook spaghetti as directed on package. Mix water and flour in medium saucepan until smooth. Stir in whipping cream and bouillon cube. Cook over low heat, stirring constantly, until mixture thickens and boils. Stir in margarine, vinegar, salt, chicken, mushrooms, and spaghetti. Season with pepper. Pour into ungreased 2-quart casserole. Sprinkle cheese on top. Bake uncovered until bubbly, about 30 minutes.

4 servings     1 serving ($\frac{1}{4}$ recipe) = 511 calories
                                     29 gm protein

# 15
## FISH

BAKED FISH · CRUSTY BAKED FISH · CHEESE FISH BAKE ·
BARBECUE BAKED FISH · SWEET AND SOUR FISH FILLETS ·
OVEN-POACHED HADDOCK · SAUCY FISH FILLETS · BAKED
FLOUNDER DELUXE · FISH STEAMED IN FOIL · TUNA PIE ·
CRAB AU GRATIN · SEAFOOD NEWBURG · TUNA CASSEROLE ·
TUNA A LA KING · WHITE CLAM SAUCE · SHRIMP WITH
LEMON-DILL SAUCE · SHRIMP SUPREME

# BAKED FISH

1½ pounds scrod or halibut (⅔ to 1 inch thick)
Salt and pepper to taste
½ cup milk

⅓ cup dairy sour cream
1 tablespoon margarine or butter
½ cup cracker crumbs

Heat oven to 325°. Cut fish into serving-size pieces. Place in lightly greased shallow baking dish. Season with salt and pepper. Pour milk over fish. Bake 20 to 25 minutes. Remove from oven. Spread sour cream on fish. Mix margarine and cracker crumbs and sprinkle over top. Bake 5 to 7 minutes longer, until light brown.

6 servings        1 serving (approximately 4 ounces fish with sauce)= 230 calories
30 gm protein


# CRUSTY BAKED FISH

*Be sure to eat the sauce so you benefit from all the calories.*

4 fish fillets (flounder, whitefish, carp)
3 tablespoons flour
1 teaspoon salt
¼ teaspoon white pepper
1 teaspoon onion powder

¾ teaspoon dill weed
½ cup beer
½ cup whipping cream
¼ cup margarine or butter, melted
1 cup cornflake crumbs
2 tablespoons snipped parsley

Heat oven to 350°. Place fish in single layer in greased baking dish 13½ x 9 x 2 inches. Mix flour, salt, pepper, onion powder, and dill weed; sprinkle over fish. Mix beer, cream, and margarine; stir in cornflake crumbs and spoon over fish. Sprinkle with parsley. Bake 30 minutes, until fish flakes easily with fork and is brown.

4 servings        1 serving (1 fillet) = 495 calories
33 gm protein

# CHEESE FISH BAKE

*Just add a salad for a quick, easy meal.*

1 cup uncooked elbow macaroni
¼ cup chopped onion
2 tablespoons margarine or butter
1 can (10½ ounces) condensed cream
  of celery or mushroom soup
½ cup milk

1 cup shredded sharp Cheddar
  cheese
1 can (8 ounces) salmon or 1 can (7
  ounces) tuna, drained and
  flaked
1 tablespoon margarine or butter
2 tablespoons bread crumbs

Heat oven to 350°. Cook macaroni as directed on package. Turn into ungreased 1½-quart casserole. Cook and stir onion in 2 tablespoons margarine until tender. Stir in soup, milk, ¾ cup of the cheese, and the tuna. Pour over macaroni and stir. Melt 1 tablespoon margarine and mix with bread crumbs. Sprinkle bread crumbs and remaining cheese on casserole. Bake 30 minutes until bubbly and light brown. Garnish with parsley if desired.

4 servings      1 serving (¼ recipe) = 455 calories
                                    26 gm protein


# BARBECUE BAKED FISH

1 pound fish fillets (thaw if frozen)
Salt and freshly ground pepper
1 tablespoon margarine or butter
4 thin slices lemon

4 thin onion rings
2 tablespoons snipped parsley
1 can (10¾ ounces) condensed
  tomato soup

Heat oven to 350°. Arrange fish in ungreased baking dish 10 x 6 x 2 inches. Season with salt and pepper. Dot with margarine and top with lemon slices, onion rings, and parsley. Bake 15 minutes. Pour soup over fish, stirring soup and fish liquid in baking dish. Bake 10 minutes longer or until fish flakes easily with fork. Stir liquid in baking dish before serving.

4 servings      1 serving (4 ounces fish with sauce) = 240 calories
                                              35 gm protein

# SWEET AND SOUR FISH FILLETS

*A new taste treat for fish.*

1½ pounds fish fillets (thaw if
    frozen)
½ cup soy sauce
1 tablespoon brown sugar
2 tablespoons vegetable oil

1 tablespoon vinegar
½ teaspoon ginger
1 clove garlic, crushed
1 tablespoon snipped parsley

Cut fish into serving pieces. Place in baking dish 10 x 6 x 2 inches.
Mix soy sauce, sugar, oil, vinegar, ginger, and garlic; pour over fish.
Let stand 20 minutes, turning fish once.

    Set oven control at broil or 550°. Drain fish, reserving marinade;
place on rack in broiler pan. Broil fish 5 inches from heat 4 minutes.
Turn, basting fish with marinade; broil 4 minutes longer or until
fish flakes easily with fork. Garnish with parsley.

6 servings      1 serving (4 ounces) = 220 calories
                                    36 gm protein


# OVEN-POACHED HADDOCK

*Prepare in the morning and pop in the oven at dinner time.*

1½ pounds haddock fillets
Juice of 1 lemon
1 bay leaf
1 tablespoon finely chopped onion
1 teaspoon snipped parsley

½ teaspoon thyme
½ teaspoon chervil
½ teaspoon sugar
3 medium tomatoes, sliced
Salt and freshly ground pepper

Cut fish into 4 serving pieces and place in ungreased baking dish
13½ x 9 x 2 inches. Mix remaining ingredients except tomatoes and
salt and pepper; pour over fish. Cover and refrigerate 3 to 4 hours.

    Heat oven to 350°. Arrage tomato slices on fish and season with
salt and pepper. Cover and bake until fish flakes easily with fork,
about 40 minutes.

4 servings      1 serving (6 ounces) = 180 calories
                                    34 gm protein

# SAUCY FISH FILLETS

1 pound fish fillets (thaw if frozen)
Dash freshly ground pepper
1 can (10½ ounces) condensed cream
    of celery soup

½ cup shredded process American
    cheese
Paprika

Heat oven to 350°. Arrange fish in shallow baking dish 10 x 6 x 2 inches. Season with pepper. Bake 15 minutes. Pour soup over fish, stirring soup and liquid in baking dish. Sprinkle cheese and paprika over fish. Bake 10 minutes longer or until fish flakes easily with fork. Stir liquid in baking dish. Garnish with parsley or lemon wedges if desired.

4 servings      1 serving (4 ounces fish with sauce) = 270 calories
                                35 gm protein

# BAKED FLOUNDER DELUXE

1 pound fresh or thawed flounder
    fillets
½ cup dairy sour cream
2 tablespoons lemon juice
1 tablespoon milk or water
1 teaspoon salt

1 teaspoon snipped chives
½ teaspoon white pepper
1½ cups cornflake crumbs
1 tablespoon Parmesan cheese
1 teaspoon salt

Heat oven to 450°. Cut fish into serving pieces if necessary. Mix sour cream, lemon juice, milk, 1 teaspoon salt, the chives, and white pepper in flat bowl. Mix cornflake crumbs, cheese, and 1 teaspoon salt. Dip fish into sour cream mixture to coat both sides, then into crumb mixture. Place in greased baking pan 15½ x 10½ x 1 inch. Bake 12 minutes.

Set oven control at broil or 550°. Broil 4 inches from heat 3 to 4 minutes until brown. Garnish with slivered almonds and snipped parsley.

4 servings      1 serving (4 ounces fish with topping) = 350 calories
                                38 gm protein

# FISH STEAMED IN FOIL

*Cooking in foil helps eliminate cooking odors.*

4-ounce fish fillet (sole, flounder, ocean perch)
1 tablespoon Creole Sauce (see page 204)
2 slices sweet Spanish onion
1 carrot, cut lengthwise in half
$\frac{1}{2}$ tomato, peeled
Salt and pepper

Heat oven to 350°. Tear piece of heavy-duty aluminum foil twice the width of fish. Place fish in center of foil. Spread Creole Sauce on fish; top with onion, carrot, and tomato, and season with salt and pepper. Bring edges of foil together and fold over twice, making a tightly locked fold. Fold each end the same way. Bake 20 minutes, until fish flakes easily with fork. To serve, fold back foil to form a dish.

1 serving
1 serving = 210 calories
34 gm protein


# TUNA PIE

*Colorful, easy-to-eat, and very good.*

1 can (6$\frac{1}{2}$ ounces) tuna, drained
1 cup shredded process sharp American cheese
1 package (3 ounces) cream cheese, cut up
$\frac{1}{4}$ cup sliced green onion
1 jar (2 ounces) shopped pimiento, drained
2 cups milk
1 cup Bisquick® buttermilk baking mix
4 eggs
$\frac{3}{4}$ teaspoon salt
Dash nutmeg

Heat oven to 400°. Grease 10-inch pie pan. Mix tuna, cheeses, onion, and pimiento in pie pan. Measure remaining ingredients into blender container; blend on high speed 15 seconds or beat ingredients 1 minute with beater. Pour over ingredients in pie pan. Bake 35 to 40 minutes, until knife inserted between center and edge comes out clean. Cool 5 minutes. Nice served with sliced tomatoes.

6 to 8 servings
$\frac{1}{6}$ pie = 350 calories
23 gm protein

## VARIATION

» *Seafood Pie:* Substitute 1 package (6 ounces) frozen crabmeat and/or shrimp, thawed and drained, for the tuna.

# CRAB AU GRATIN

*A tasty, soft casserole.*

1 package (6 ounces) frozen crab-
    meat, thawed
2 tablespoons margarine or butter
3 tablespoons flour
½ teaspoon salt
⅛ teaspoon paprika
½ cup milk
½ cup half-and-half

¼ cup white wine
½ cup shredded Cheddar cheese
1 can (2 ounces) sliced mushrooms,
    drained
1½ teaspoons snipped chives or
    green onion
2½ tablespoons bread crumbs

Heat oven to 400°. Drain crabmeat, reserving liquid. Melt margarine in saucepan over low heat. Stir in flour, salt, and paprika. Cook
over low heat, stirring until smooth and bubbly. Stir in milk, half-
and-half, wine, and reserved crab liquid. Heat to boiling, stirring
constantly. Boil and stir 1 minute. Reduce heat; stir in cheese, mushrooms, and chives. Fold in crabmeat. Turn into greased 1-quart casserole. Sprinkle bread crumbs on top. Bake 15 minutes until top is
golden brown.

3 or 4 servings    1 serving (¼ recipe) = 245 calories
                            14 gm protein

# SEAFOOD NEWBURG

1 package (6 ounces) frozen crab-
    meat and/or shrimp, thawed
¼ cup margarine or butter
2 tablespoons flour
½ teaspoon salt
⅛ teaspoon nutmeg
⅛ teaspoon cayenne pepper

2 cups half-and-half
3 egg yolks
1 tablespoon plus 1½ teaspoons dry
    sherry
Hot cooked rice
Snipped parsley

Drain crabmeat and shrimp, reserving liquid. Melt margarine in
saucepan. Stir in flour, salt, nutmeg, and cayenne pepper. Cook
over low heat, stirring constantly until smooth and bubbly. Stir in
half-and-half. Heat to boiling, stirring constantly. Boil and stir 1
minute. Beat egg yolks slightly; stir small amount of hot sauce into
them; then stir yolks into hot mixture in saucepan. Stir in crabmeat
and shrimp and reserved liquid. Heat, stirring constantly, until hot
and thickened. Remove from heat; stir in sherry. Serve over rice,
garnished with parsley.

4 or 5 servings    1 serving (⅕ recipe) = 300 calories
                            12 gm protein

# TUNA CASSEROLE

1 can (10½ ounces) condensed cream of celery, chicken, or mushroom soup
¼ cup milk

1 can (7 ounces) tuna, drained and flaked
3 hard-cooked eggs, sliced
1 cup peas
1 cup crushed potato chips

Heat oven to 350°. Blend soup and milk in ungreased 1-quart casserole. Stir in tuna, eggs, and peas, and sprinkle with potato chips. Bake 30 minutes or until bubbly.

4 servings    1 serving (¼ casserole) = 300 calories
                                      23 gm protein


# TUNA A LA KING

½ cup chopped celery
2 tablespoons chopped onion
1 tablespoon margarine or butter
1 can (10½ ounces) condensed cream of mushroom soup
½ cup milk

1 can (7 ounces) tuna, drained and flaked
2 tablespoons chopped pimiento
4 slices toast
Snipped parsley

Cook and stir celery and onion in margarine until tender. Blend in soup and milk. Stir in tuna and pimiento. Heat, stirring constantly, just to simmering. Reduce heat and simmer 5 minutes, stirring frequently. Serve on toast and garnish with parsley.

4 servings    1 serving (¼ recipe) = 250 calories
                                   19 gm protein

# WHITE CLAM SAUCE

*Pasta in lots of sauce will easily go down.*

1 clove garlic, minced
½ cup olive oil
2 tablespoons snipped parsley
¼ teaspoon crushed red peppers, optional

1 can (10¼ ounces) whole baby clams, drained
Hot cooked spaghetti, ¼ cup per serving

Cook and stir garlic in olive oil. Stir in parsley, red peppers, and clams. Heat to boiling; reduce heat, and simmer 3 minutes. Serve over spaghetti.

3 servings        1 serving (approximately ⅓ cup sauce) = 416 calories
                                                            15 gm protein

NOTE: For red clam sauce, heat clams in marinara sauce.


# SHRIMP WITH LEMON-DILL SAUCE

*Quick to fix, with a snappy taste.*

1 pound deveined and shelled medium shrimp
2 green onions, thinly sliced
¼ cup margarine or butter

1 tablespoon snipped fresh dill or 1 teaspoon dried dill weed
2 tablespoons lemon juice
Salt and freshly ground pepper

Thaw shrimp if frozen. Cook shrimp and onion in margarine in large skillet, stirring frequently, 5 minutes, or until shrimp are pink and firm and onion is tender. Add dill and lemon juice; season with salt and pepper, and toss.

4 servings        1 serving (¼ recipe) = 250 calories
                                          28 gm protein

# SHRIMP SUPREME

*Even kids love shrimp cooked this way.*

1 small onion, chopped
2 tablespoons chopped green
   pepper
2 tablespoons margarine or butter
2 tablespoons flour
½ teaspoon salt
1 cup water
¼ cup tomato juice

Dash pepper sauce
1 teaspoon Worcestershire sauce
1 cup shredded process American
   cheese
1 pound cleaned cooked shrimp
   (fresh or frozen)
3 cups hot cooked rice

Cook and stir onion and green pepper in margarine until tender. Stir in flour and salt. Cook and stir until bubbly. Stir in water, tomato juice, pepper sauce, and Worcestershire sauce. Heat to boiling, stirring constantly. Boil and stir 1 minute. Stir in cheese and shrimp. Heat until cheese is melted. Serve over rice.

4 servings     1 serving (¼ recipe) = 490 calories
                                 38 gm protein

# *16*

## *MAIN DISH SAUCES*

SAUCERY · TANGY CHEESE SAUCE FOR FISH · HERB-CHEESE
SAUCE · CUMBERLAND SAUCE · PARSLEY-WINE SAUCE ·
SWEDISH SAUCE · CREOLE SAUCE · MUSTARD SAUCE ·
MORNAY SAUCE · CREAM SAUCE · BORDELAISE SAUCE ·
BLENDER BEARNAISE SAUCE · BLENDER HOLLANDAISE
SAUCE · BASIC BROWN SAUCE · CREAMY GIBLET GRAVY ·
QUICK ONION GRAVY · GRAVY IN A HURRY · WHITE SAUCE ·
VEGETABLE TOPPING

# SAUCERY

Lucky the homemaker who discovers the versatile sauces always on hand in cans of condensed soup. Whether you're adding new flavor appeal to leftover meat or preparing gravy for a chicken, a can of soup is ready to fill your sauce-making needs with ease.

White sauce or cream sauce comes all blended for you in a can of cream soup. Whenever a recipe calls for white sauce, choose the one with the special flavor you want—cream of chicken, mushroom, or celery soup. Simply add a little liquid to thin the soup-sauce to the thickness you prefer, and use it as a pour-on cream sauce.

Gravy is always available in the cream soups. Just blend with a little liquid and/or drippings for the kind of gravy your family will applaud.

A can of condensed soup is an ever-ready kitchen help—whether you use it for white sauce in a casserole or as cooking liquid in a stew. Here are some suggestions for creating your own recipes with condensed soups.

## USE A CAN OF SOUP FOR

### Tomato Sauce

Heat 1 can of cream of tomato soup. For a thinner sauce, add milk or water to achieve desired consistency. Season with Worcestershire sauce, prepared mustard, horseradish, or herbs. Good for hamburgers, pork chops, and other meats.

### Gravy

Stir 1 can cream soup or golden mushroom soup into 2 to 3 tablespoons meat drippings. Add about $\frac{1}{4}$ cup water if you like thinner gravy.

### White Sauce, Cream Sauce

Heat 1 can cream soup or Cheddar cheese soup and $\frac{1}{4}$ to $\frac{1}{2}$ cup water, stirring constantly, for medium white sauce—so easy for creamed chicken or vegetables. This amount is adequate for $\frac{1}{2}$ to 1 cup diced or chopped meat, fish, seafood, or 4 sliced hard-cooked eggs. One can of soup also provides a ready-made sauce for 1 pound meat or fish, 2 pounds chicken parts, 2 cups cooked vegetables, 6 chops, or 4 to 6 sandwiches.

### Casseroles

Heat 1 can cream, Cheddar cheese, or tomato soup and $\frac{1}{4}$ cup water or milk. This makes sauce for about 2 cups macaroni or noodles or $1\frac{1}{2}$ cups cooked rice. Enhance casseroles with seasonings and cooked meat or vegetables.

### Meat Stock or Broth

Condensed beef broth, chicken broth, or consommé can be substituted for homemade stock. Excellent for many stews and pot roasts.

### Chicken Stew

Cream soups, chicken broth, or chicken soups can be used for part of cooking water. When using a vegetable soup or one with noodles or rice, add during the last 5 to 10 minutes.

### Meat Stew, Pot Roast

Consommé, beef broth, chicken broth, golden mushroom, or tomato soup can be used for part of the liquid to cook meat. For vegetables in stew, stir in vegetable soups during the last 5 to 10 minutes.

### Homemade Soup

Canned soups add flavor and body to homemade soup.

| Sauce | For | Use 1 can | Directions |
|---|---|---|---|
| *Almond* | Chicken, veal, seafood | Cream of chicken or Cream of mushroom | Cook and stir 1 tablespoon minced onion in 1 teaspoon margarine or butter. Stir in soup, $\frac{1}{3}$ cup water, $\frac{1}{4}$ cup chopped almonds. Add extra interest with 1 tablespoon sherry. |
| *Creamy cheese* | Vegetables, chicken | Cream of celery | Blend 1 package (3 ounces) cream cheese, softened, into soup. Stir in $\frac{1}{4}$ to $\frac{1}{3}$ cup milk and heat, stirring constantly. |
| *Curry* | Chicken, veal, lamb, seafood | Cream of asparagus or Cream of celery or Cream of chicken | Heat soup, $\frac{1}{4}$ to $\frac{1}{3}$ cup milk, and $\frac{1}{4}$ to $\frac{1}{2}$ teaspoon curry powder, stirring constantly. |
| *Herb* | Chicken, fish, vegetables, veal, eggs | Cream of celery or Cream of chicken or Cream of mushroom | Heat soup, $\frac{1}{4}$ to $\frac{1}{2}$ cup milk, and dash basil, marjoram, poultry seasoning, sage, or thyme, stirring constantly. |
| *Nut* | Chicken, veal, vegetables | Cream of mushroom | Heat soup, $\frac{1}{4}$ to $\frac{1}{2}$ cup milk and $\frac{1}{4}$ cup chopped walnuts, stirring constantly. |
| *Parsley* | Fish, eggs, vegetables | Cream of celery | Heat soup, $\frac{1}{4}$ to $\frac{1}{3}$ cup milk, and 1 tablespoon snipped parsley, stirring constantly. |
| *Pimiento-Egg* | Fish | Cream of celery | Cook and stir 1 tablespoon minced onion in 1 teaspoon margarine until tender. Stir in soup and $\frac{1}{3}$ cup water. Heat, stirring constantly. |

# TANGY CHEESE SAUCE FOR FISH

$\frac{1}{4}$ cup chopped celery
1 small clove garlic, minced
$\frac{1}{8}$ teaspoon dry mustard
2 tablespoons margarine or butter

1 can (10$\frac{1}{2}$ ounces) condensed
   Cheddar cheese soup
$\frac{1}{3}$ cup milk
1 tablespoon chopped dill pickle

Cook and stir celery, garlic, and mustard in margarine until celery is tender. Stir in soup and milk. Heat, stirring constantly, just to simmering. Reduce heat and simmer 5 minutes. Stir in pickle.

1½ cups sauce    ¼ cup = 100 calories
                          2 gm protein

## HERB-CHEESE SAUCE

*Add extra protein to vegetables.*

1 can (10½ ounces) condensed cream
   of mushroom soup
⅓ to ½ cup milk
1 cup shredded Cheddar cheese (4
   ounces)

1 tablespoon snipped parsley
Generous dash tarragon leaves,
   crushed

Blend soup and milk in small saucepan. Stir in remaining ingredients. Heat, stirring constantly, just to simmering. Reduce heat and simmer 5 minutes. Serve over cooked peas and onions, green beans, or broccoli.

2 cups sauce    ¼ cup = 100 calories
                          5 gm protein

## CUMBERLAND SAUCE

1 cup currant jelly
½ cup Madeira wine
¼ cup shredded orange peel
1 tablespoon shredded lemon peel
1 small piece crystallized, chopped

ginger, or ground ginger to
   taste
½ teaspoon dry mustard
Dash cayenne red pepper

Melt jelly in small saucepan over low heat. Stir in remaining ingredients. Serve warm or cold with meat.

1½ cups    ¼ cup = 160 calories
                     0 protein

# PARSLEY-WINE SAUCE

1 tablespoon finely chopped onion
⅓ cup dry white wine
3 tablespoons margarine or butter

1 tablespoon snipped parsley
2 drops pepper sauce
Freshly ground pepper

Cook onion and wine uncovered in small saucepan until wine is reduced in half. Stir in margarine, parsley, and pepper sauce. Season with pepper. Serve on steak, chicken, or pasta.

About ⅓ cup     ⅓ cup = 210 calories
                    1 gm protein


# SWEDISH SAUCE

*A tangy, high-calorie accompaniment for cold meat.*

1 cup mayonnaise
½ cup unsweetened applesauce

1 tablespoon grated horseradish
Freshly ground pepper

Mix all ingredients; cover and refrigerate. Serve with cold meat.

1½ cups     ¼ cup = 270 calories
                  ½ gm protein


# CREOLE SAUCE

*A colorful, tasty sauce*

1 small green pepper, sliced
1 small onion, sliced
½ cup sliced fresh mushrooms or 1 can (4 ounces) sliced mushrooms, drained

2 tablespoons margarine or butter
1 can (10¾ ounces) condensed tomato soup
¼ cup water
1 teaspoon vinegar

Cook and stir green pepper, onion, and mushrooms in margarine until vegetables are tender. Stir in soup, water, and vinegar. Heat, stirring constantly, just to simmering. Reduce heat and simmer 5 minutes. Serve over omelet, hamburgers, or baked fish.

2 cups sauce     ½ cup = 65 calories
                    1 gm protein

# MUSTARD SAUCE

Heat 1 cup dairy cream and $\frac{1}{4}$ to $\frac{1}{2}$ cup spicy prepared mustard in small saucepan, stirring constantly, until mixture is smooth and hot.

About 1 cup      $\frac{1}{4}$ cup = 150 calories
3 gm protein

# MORNAY SAUCE

1 can (10$\frac{3}{4}$ ounces) condensed cream
   of mushroom soup
$\frac{1}{2}$ cup shredded Swiss cheese

$\frac{1}{3}$ cup light cream (20%) or milk
2 tablespoons grated Parmesan
   cheese

Heat all ingredients, stirring constantly, just to simmering. Reduce heat; simmer 5 minutes. Serve over cooked meats, poultry, fish, vegetables, or poached eggs.

1$\frac{1}{2}$ cups sauce      $\frac{1}{4}$ cup = 125 calories
5 gm protein

# CREAM SAUCE

1 can (10$\frac{1}{2}$ ounces) condensed cream
   of celery, chicken, or mushroom
   soup

$\frac{1}{4}$ to $\frac{1}{2}$ cup milk

Heat soup and milk, stirring constantly, just to simmering. Reduce heat; simmer about 5 minutes, stirring frequently. Use for creamed vegetables and meats.

About 1 to 1$\frac{1}{2}$ cups      $\frac{1}{4}$ cup = 85 calories
2 gm protein

### VARIATIONS

» *Instant Cheese Sauce:* Substitute 1 can (10$\frac{3}{4}$) ounces condensed Cheddar cheese soup for the cream soup.

» *Special Cheese Sauce:* Use any of the condensed cream soups and add $\frac{1}{2}$ cup shredded Cheddar cheese before heating to simmering.

# BORDELAISE SAUCE

1 teaspoon margarine or butter
1 teaspoon chopped onion
1 mushroom, chopped

$\frac{1}{4}$ cup Basic Brown Sauce (page 207)
$\frac{1}{4}$ cup red wine

Melt margarine in small skillet; cook and stir onion and mushroom in margarine until onion is tender. Remove from heat.

Heat Basic Brown Sauce, stirring frequently, until sauce is reduced by half. Stir in wine, onion, and mushroom; simmer 2 to 3 minutes. Serve with beef.

$\frac{1}{3}$ cup    $\frac{1}{3}$ cup = 240 calories
                        1 gm protein

# BLENDER BEARNAISE SAUCE

1 tablespoon dry white wine
2 teaspoons tarragon vinegar
$\frac{1}{2}$ teaspoon lemon juice
$\frac{1}{2}$ teaspoon bottled meat glaze

2 egg yolks
$\frac{3}{4}$ cup margarine or butter (1$\frac{1}{2}$ sticks)
1 tablespoon snipped chives

Place wine, vinegar, lemon juice, meat glaze, and egg yolks in blender; mix at high speed 5 seconds.

Heat margarine over low heat until melted and bubbly. Adding hot margarine slowly to egg yolk mixture, blend at medium speed until sauce is smooth. Mix in chives at low speed. Serve at room temperature.

About 1 cup sauce    $\frac{1}{4}$ cup = 335 calories
                        2 gm protein

# BLENDER HOLLANDAISE SAUCE

4 egg yolks
2 to 3 tablespoons lemon juice
$\frac{1}{4}$ teaspoon salt

Dash pepper
$\frac{1}{2}$ cup margarine or butter, melted

Place egg yolk, lemon juice, salt, and pepper in blender. Mix at high speed and slowly pour warm margarine into egg yolks. Blend 1 minute. Serve immediately.

About 1 cup sauce    $\frac{1}{4}$ cup = 265 calories
                        3 gm protein

# BASIC BROWN SAUCE

2 teaspoons margarine or butter  $\frac{2}{3}$ cup beef broth
2 teaspoons flour

Melt margarine in saucepan over low heat. Blend in flour. Cook over low heat, stirring until mixture is smooth and bubbly. Increase heat to medium, and cook and stir until mixture is brown. Remove from heat; stir in beef broth. Heat to boiling, stirring constantly. Boil and stir 1 minute. Refrigerate or freeze until ready to use.

About $\frac{2}{3}$ cup  $\frac{1}{3}$ cup = 115 calories
1 gm protein

# CREAMY GIBLET GRAVY

Giblets from chicken, cooked and
  finely chopped
$\frac{1}{2}$ cup chopped celery
2 tablespoons margarine or butter

1 can (10$\frac{1}{2}$ ounces) condensed cream
  of chicken soup
$\frac{1}{3}$ cup water

Cook and stir giblets and celery in margarine until giblets are brown and celery is tender. Stir in soup and water. Heat, stirring constantly, just to simmering. Reduce heat and simmer 5 minutes, stirring frequently.

2 cups gravy  $\frac{1}{4}$ cup = 70 calories
2 gm protein

# QUICK ONION GRAVY

1 cup sliced onion
1 small clove garlic, minced
3 tablespoons margarine or butter

1 can (10$\frac{1}{2}$ ounces) condensed
  golden mushroom soup
$\frac{1}{2}$ cup water

Cook and stir onion and garlic in margarine until onion is tender. Stir in soup and water. Heat, stirring constantly, just to simmering. Reduce heat; simmer 5 minutes, stirring frequently. Serve on beef patties or sliced cooked beef or pork.

About 1$\frac{1}{2}$ cups gravy  $\frac{1}{4}$ cup = 100 calories
1 gm protein

# GRAVY IN A HURRY

2 to 4 tablespoons pan drippings
$\frac{1}{4}$ to $\frac{1}{3}$ cup water
1 can (10$\frac{1}{2}$ ounces) cream soup,

celery, chicken, mushroom,
golden mushroom

Remove meat from pan. Pour off drippings, and measure 2 to 4 tablespoons back into pan. Stir in $\frac{1}{4}$ to $\frac{1}{3}$ cup water, loosening brown bits on pan bottom. Stir in soup. Heat, stirring constantly, just to simmering. Reduce heat and simmer 5 minutes, stirring frequently. Serve with fried chicken, roast beef, roast pork, pork chops, hamburgers, or baked ham.

1$\frac{1}{2}$ cups gravy     $\frac{1}{4}$ cup = 95 calories
                    $\frac{1}{2}$ gm protein


# WHITE SAUCE

$\frac{1}{2}$ cup water
2 tablespoons flour
$\frac{1}{2}$ cup whipping cream

$\frac{1}{4}$ teaspoon salt
$\frac{1}{8}$ teaspoon white pepper
2 tablespoons margarine or butter

Mix water and flour in small saucepan until smooth. Stir in cream, salt, and pepper. Cook over low heat, stirring constantly, until mixture thickens and boils. Boil and stir 1 minute. Stir in margarine.

About 1 cup     $\frac{1}{4}$ cup = 70 calories
                    $\frac{1}{2}$ gm protein


VARIATION
» *Thin White Sauce:* Decrease flour to 1 tablespoon.

NOTE: Cover sauce with waxed paper to prevent "skin" from forming. Mixture will thicken on standing. Add $\frac{1}{4}$ to $\frac{1}{2}$ cup water or cream for a thinner consistency.

# VEGETABLE TOPPING

1 can ($10\frac{3}{4}$ ounces) condensed
    Cheddar cheese soup
$\frac{1}{4}$ cup milk

$\frac{1}{4}$ teaspoon prepared mustard
1 hard-cooked egg, sliced

Heat soup, milk, and mustard, stirring constantly, just to simmering. Stir in egg slices. Reduce heat and simmer about 5 minutes.

$1\frac{1}{2}$ cups sauce      $\frac{1}{4}$ cup = 75 calories
                      4 gm protein

# 17

## *DESSERTS*

ICED FRUIT · MACEDOINE OF FRUIT · TROPICAL FRUIT AND
WINE COMPOTE · BANANA IN SHERRY · RASPBERRY MELON
BOATS · MINTED PINAPPLE · APPLESAUCE DELUXE · FRUIT
SHERBET · SPRING DELIGHT · BROILED GRAPEFRUIT ·
STRAWBERRY SHERBET · RICH LEMON SHERBET ·
RASPBERRY-PINEAPPLE ICE · PEACH MELBA · PEANUT
BUTTER ICE CREAM BALLS · APPLE SOUFFLE · CHEESE POT
DE CREME · PINEAPPLE CREAM · FROSTY LEMONADE FLUFF ·
CREAMY RICE PUDDING · OLD-FASHIONED RICE PUDDING ·
CHANTILLY MELBA · NUT BARS · PEANUT BUTTER COOKIES ·
CREPES SUZETTE · CREPES · CHOCOLATE MOUSSE PIE ·
PECAN PIE · STRAWBERRY-YOGURT REFRIGERATOR PIE ·
APPLESAUCE CAKE · BOURBON POUND CAKE · RUM CAKE ·
LEMON POUND CAKE · CARROT CAKE · GINGERBREAD ·
PASTRY FOR 8 OR 9 INCH ONE-CRUST PIE

# ICED FRUIT

1 cup fruit cocktail
½ cup cut-up fresh fruit

1 tablespoon crème de menthe

Place fruit in small bowl, sprinkle crème de menthe over it, and toss. Put in freezer and stir occasionally, until chilled, 40 to 50 minutes.

2 servings        1 serving (about ¾ cup) = 150 calories
                                              0 gm protein

# MACEDOINE OF FRUIT

2 red apples
2 pears
1 pineapple, pared, cored, and cut
   into spears
2 grapefruit, pared and sectioned
4 oranges, pared and sectioned

Seedless green grapes and Tokay
   grapes
1 cup currant jelly
2 tablespoons orange juice
¼ cup Galliano liqueur

Slice unpared apples and pears into large bowl. Add remaining fruits.

Melt jelly in small saucepan over low heat, stirring constantly. Remove from heat; stir in orange juice and liqueur. Pour sauce over fruit, carefully lifting fruit with fork so that all pieces will be glazed.

6 to 8 servings        1 serving (about 1⅓ cups) = 350 calories
                                                    2 gm protein

NOTE: If desired, dessert can be prepared ahead. Dip apple and pear slices into lemon or lime juice. Cover bowl of fruit and refrigerate. Glaze can be refrigerated and heated at serving time.

# TROPICAL FRUIT AND WINE COMPOTE

1 can (13½ ounces) pineapple
   chunks, drained
1 medium grapefruit, pared and
   sectioned
2 small bananas, sliced

1 cup seeded Malaga grapes
¼ cup sugar
⅓ cup sherry
2 tablespoons Madeira wine

Gently mix fruit, sugar, and wine. Cover and refrigerate. Top with whipped cream.

6 servings      1 serving (about $\frac{3}{4}$ cup) = 160 calories
                                            1 gm protein


## BANANA IN SHERRY

1 firm banana
1 tablespoon margarine or butter

1 tablespoon plus 1$\frac{1}{2}$ teaspoons
    honey
2 teaspoons sherry or red wine

Cut banana lengthwise into 4 pieces, then crosswise into 2-inch pieces. Melt margarine in skillet; cook banana in margarine until golden. Add honey and stir gently to coat banana pieces. Cook over low heat 2 to 3 minutes. Remove from heat, add sherry, and heat 1 to 2 minutes. Serve warm or cold.

1 serving      1 serving = 340 calories
                              2 gm protein


## RASPBERRY MELON BOATS

1 package (10 ounces) frozen rasp-
    berries, thawed
1 tablespoon sugar
1 tablespoon cornstarch

$\frac{1}{2}$ cup orange juice
1 small cantaloupe
1 cup raspberry ice

Drain raspberries and reserve $\frac{1}{2}$ cup syrup. Mix sugar and cornstarch in small saucepan. Stir in reserved syrup and the orange juice. Cook, stirring constantly, until mixture thickens and boils. Cool.

Stir in raspberries. Cut cantaloupe into quarters. Remove seeds and rind. Place scoop of ice in each quarter. Spoon raspberry sauce on ice.

4 servings      1 serving = 180 calories
                              2 gm protein

VARIATION

» Vanilla ice cream can be substituted for the raspberry ice.

# MINTED PINEAPPLE

2 cans (13½ ounces each) pineapple
   chunks, drained

3 tablespoons white crème de
   menthe
3 tablespoons snipped mint

Divide pineapple chunks among 4 dessert dishes. Drizzle with crème de menthe and sprinkle with mint.

4 servings      1 serving (about ¾ cup) = 150 calories
                                     1 gm protein


# APPLESAUCE DELUXE

1 jar (24 ounces) sweetened
   applesauce
¼ cup sugar

½ cup toasted almonds, chopped
½ cup white wine, optional
½ cup dairy sour cream

Mix all ingredients; cover and refrigerate.

8 servings      1 serving (a generous half cup) = 200 calories
                                             2 gm protein


# FRUIT SHERBET

½ cup whipping cream
½ can (6-ounce size) frozen orange
   juice concentrate, partially
   thawed

1 ripe medium banana, cut into
   pieces
1 can (13½ ounces) pineapple
   chunks, frozen and partially
   thawed

Place whipping cream, orange juice concentrate, and banana pieces in blender. Cut pineapple chunks into pieces; place in blender. Cover and blend at high speed until smooth. Pour into 8″ or 9″ square baking or bread pan. Cover and freeze until firm.

4 servings      1 cup = 240 calories
                    2 gm protein

# SPRING DELIGHT

2 cups fresh strawberries          4 splits champagne, chilled
2 tablespoons sugar

Sprinkle strawberries with sugar and divide among 4 goblets. Pour champagne over each and serve immediately.

4 servings          1 serving = 180 calories
                              1 gm protein

# BROILED GRAPEFRUIT

1 medium grapefruit          Margarine or butter
2 tablespoons brown sugar or
   honey

Cut grapefruit in half; remove seeds. Cut around edges and membranes of halves to loosen fruit; remove centers. Sprinkle sugar on halves and dot with margarine.

Set oven control at broil or 550°. Place halves in shallow baking pan. Broil 4 to 6 inches from heat until juice bubbles and edge of peel turns light brown, about 8 minutes. Serve hot.

2 servings          $\frac{1}{2}$ grapefruit = 155 calories
                              1 gm protein

# STRAWBERRY SHERBET

1 package (10 ounces) frozen straw-          1 can (6 ounces) evaporated milk
   berries, partially thawed                 $\frac{1}{2}$ cup sugar
1 tablespoon lemon juice                     Few drops red food color, optional
1 cup crushed ice

Break strawberries into chunks. Place all ingredients in blender. Cover and blend at high speed until smooth and thick, 2 minutes. Pour into 8″ or 9″ baking or bread pan  Cover and freeze until firm.

4 servings          1 serving ($\frac{3}{4}$ cup) = 235 calories
                              3 gm protein

# RICH LEMON SHERBET

1 cup sugar
1 pint whipping cream
½ cup lemon juice

Few drops yellow food color,
  optional

Mix sugar and cream until sugar is dissolved. Stir in lemon juice and food color. Pour into 8-inch square pan or divide mixture among 8 sherbet dishes. Freeze 3 hours, until firm. Remove from freezer 5 minutes before serving.

8 servings    1 serving (about ½ cup) = 275 calories
                                          1 gm protein

# RASPBERRY-PINEAPPLE ICE

1 package (10 ounces) frozen
  raspberries

1 can (13½ ounces) frozen pineapple
  chunks
½ cup whipped cream

Break frozen fruits apart with fork. Place fruits, a small amount at a time, in blender; blend at high speed until smooth. Serve immediately, or pour into 8″ or 9″ square baking or bread pan, and freeze for a short time. Top with whipped cream.

4 servings    1 serving (about ¾ cup) = 240 calories
                                          2 gm protein

NOTE: Serve this ice in meringue shells for a party dessert.

# PEACH MELBA

1 pint raspberries or 1 package (10
  ounces) frozen raspberries,
  thawed
1 jar (8 ounces) currant jelly

1 pint vanilla ice cream
2 large peaches, peeled and cut
  into halves, or 4 canned peach
  halves

Press raspberries and jelly through sieve; stir until smooth. Put ½ cup ice cream in each of 4 dessert dishes. Place peach half, cut side down, on ice cream. Drizzle raspberry sauce on each.

4 servings    1 serving = 440 calories
                           4 gm protein

# PEANUT BUTTER ICE CREAM BALLS

1 cup graham cracker crumbs
¼ cup peanut butter
2 tablespoons sugar
¼ teaspoon cinnamon

1 quart vanilla ice cream
Chocolate syrup or thin fudge
sauce

Mix crumbs, peanut butter, sugar, and cinnamon. Scoop ice cream into 8 balls. Roll balls in crumb mixture, place in baking pan, and freeze. Serve with chocolate syrup.

8 servings     1 ice cream ball = 290 calories
6 gm protein

# APPLE SOUFFLE

*Easy and light.*

1 egg white
⅓ cup applesauce

Sugar

Heat oven to 350°. Grease 10-ounce custard cup with margarine. Beat egg white until stiff peaks form. Fold in applesauce. Turn into custard cup. Bake 35 to 40 minutes. Sprinkle sugar on top. Extra rich served with Whipped Brandy Cream (page 230).

1 soufflé = 90 calories
3 gm protein

# CHEESE POT DE CREME

4 eggs
Dash each salt, cayenne pepper,
and nutmeg

2 cups whipping cream
1½ cups shredded Swiss cheese (6 ounces)

Heat oven to 350°. Beat eggs and seasonings thoroughly with fork. Continue beating, adding cream gradually. Stir in 1 cup of the cheese. Divide mixture among 8 small pots de creme or custard cups. Place cups in pan with 1 inch of hot water. Bake 30 to 35 minutes or until knife inserted in center comes out clean. Remove from oven and sprinkle remaining cheese in cups. Serve immediately.

8 servings     1 pot = 305 calories
10 gm protein

# PINEAPPLE CREAM

1 can (8¾ ounces) crushed
    pineapple
⅓ cup uncooked regular rice
¼ teaspoon salt

2 teaspoons lemon juice
1½ cups miniature marshmallows
1 cup mandarin orange segments
1 cup chilled whipping cream

Drain pineapple, reserving juice. Measure juice; add water to make
⅔ cup. Heat pineapple liquid, rice, and salt to boiling, stirring once
or twice. Reduce heat to simmer, cover pan tightly, and cook 14
minutes. (Do not lift cover or stir.)

    Remove from heat; carefully stir in pineapple and lemon juice
and cool. Stir in marshmallows and orange segments. Beat cream in
chilled bowl until stiff. Fold into pineapple-rice mixture and
refrigerate.

6 servings     1 serving (about ¾ cup) = 225 calories
                           2 gm protein


# FROSTY LEMONADE FLUFF

2 tablespoons flour
½ cup sugar
1 cup water

¼ cup frozen lemonade concentrate
    (thawed)
2 drops yellow food color, optional
1 cup chilled whipping cream

Mix flour and sugar in small saucepan. Stir in water. Cook over
medium heat, stirring constantly, until mixture thickens and boils.
Boil and stir 1 minute. Remove from heat; stir in lemonade concentrate and food color. Press plastic wrap onto lemonade mixture in
pan to prevent "skin" from forming on top. Cool.

    Beat cream in chilled bowl until stiff. Fold in lemonade mixture.
Pour into 8" or 9" square baking or bread pan. Cover and freeze
until firm.

6 servings     1 serving (about ⅔ cup) = 215 calories
                           1 gm protein

# CREAMY RICE PUDDING

*Top with your favorite high-calorie sauce or whipped cream.*

2 cups cooked rice
2 cups milk
$\frac{1}{4}$ cup sugar

2 teaspoons margarine or butter
$\frac{1}{2}$ teaspoon cinnamon

Measure all ingredients into heavy saucepan. Cook over medium heat, stirring frequently, until thickened to desired consistency, 10 to 15 minutes. Serve warm or cold. If desired, spoon pudding into heat-proof shallow dish and place under broiler a short time, until top is golden brown.

4 servings      1 serving (about $\frac{3}{4}$ cup) = 250 calories
6 gm protein


# OLD-FASHIONED RICE PUDDING

$1\frac{3}{4}$ cups water
$\frac{1}{2}$ teaspoon salt
$\frac{1}{2}$ cup converted rice
2 cups milk
2 eggs

$\frac{1}{3}$ cup sugar
1 teaspoon vanilla
$\frac{1}{4}$ cup raisins
Nutmeg

Heat water, salt, and rice in saucepan to boiling. Reduce heat, cover, and cook 30 minutes, until all liquid is absorbed. Stir in milk; heat to boiling, stirring occasionally. Cook about 5 minutes until slightly thickened. Beat eggs; stir in sugar and vanilla. Stir in rice mixture.

Heat oven to 350°. Pour rice mixture into greased $1\frac{1}{2}$-quart casserole. Stir in raisins and sprinkle nutmeg on top. Place casserole in pan with 1 inch of hot water. Bake 45 to 50 minutes, until set. Serve warm or cold.

5 or 6 servings      1 serving (about $\frac{3}{4}$ cup) = 180 calories
6 gm protein

# CHANTILLY MELBA

1 cup chilled whipping cream
¼ cup confectioners' sugar
1 teaspoon vanilla

1 package (10 ounces) frozen raspberries, thawed
¼ cup confectioners' sugar
½ teaspoon vanilla

Beat cream, ¼ cup confectioners' sugar, and 1 teaspoon vanilla in chilled bowl until stiff.

Place raspberries, ¼ cup confectioners' sugar, and ½ teaspoon vanilla in blender. Cover and blend on high speed about 30 seconds. Fold into cream. Serve immediately in dessert dishes or pour into 8″ or 9″ square baking or bread pan, and freeze until firm.

4 servings    1 serving (about ¾ cup) = 300 calories
2 gm protein

# NUT BARS

2 cups all-purpose flour
1 cup firm margarine or butter
1 cup ground pecans or walnuts

1 tablespoon water
1 teaspoon vanilla
¾ cup confectioners' sugar

Heat oven to 375°. Measure flour into bowl; cut in margarine thoroughly. Stir in nuts, vanilla, and water. Press mixture evenly into ungreased baking pan 9 x 9 x 2 inches. Bake 20 to 25 minutes. Cool slightly. Cut into bars, 2 x 1½ inches, and roll each in confectioners' sugar.

24 bars    1 bar = 150 calories
2 gm protein

NOTE: Add a few drops of water if mixture is too dry.

# PEANUT BUTTER COOKIES

1 cup margarine or butter
1 cup chunky-style peanut butter
1 cup granulated sugar
1 cup brown sugar (packed)
2 eggs

1 teaspoon vanilla
2½ cups all-purpose flour
1 teaspoon baking powder
1 teaspoon baking soda
1 teaspoon salt

Beat margarine, peanut butter, sugars, eggs, and vanilla in large mixer bowl until smooth. Mix in flour, baking powder, baking soda, and salt with spoon. Refrigerate dough 1 hour.

Heat oven to 350°. Shape dough into 1-inch balls. Place 2 inches apart on ungreased baking sheet. Flatten with floured fork, making crisscross pattern. Bake 12 minutes or until light brown. Remove to rack and cool.

6 dozen cookies         1 cookie = 80 calories
                                    2 gm protein

» *Orange Peanut Butter Cookies:* Add 2 tablespoons grated oange peel to flour mixture.

» *Coconut Balls:* Roll balls in flaked coconut.

» *Peanut Butter Sandwich Cookies:* After baking, spread half the cookies with peanut butter; top with remaining cookies.

» *Jelly Thumbprint Cookies:* Before baking, press thumb in center of each ball. After baking, press thumb in center again, and fill indentation with jelly.

» *Peanut Butter Spritz Cookies:* Put dough through cookie press. If desired, dip ends of cookies in melted chocolate.


# CREPES SUZETTE

*A lot of work, but worth it! Delicious!*

3 Crêpes (page 222)
2 to 3 tablespoons margarine
¼ teaspoon grated orange or lemon peel
2 to 3 tablespoons orange juice

1 tablespoon sugar
1 tablespoon orange liqueur (Cointreau, curaçao, Grand Marnier)
1 tablespoon brandy
1 teaspoon sugar

Prepare crêpes as directed on page 222 or from frozen prepared batter. When removing crêpes from griddle, stack so first-baked side is down. Cool, keeping crêpes covered to prevent them from drying out. Use 3 crêpes for this recipe. Remaining crêpes can be stacked with waxed paper between, wrapped in aluminum foil, and frozen.

In small skillet, heat margarine, orange peel and juice, and 1 tablespoon sugar to boiling, stirring occasionally. Cook 1 minute.

Fold crêpes into fourths; place in hot orange·sauce, and turn once. Sprinkle with 1 teaspoon sugar. Heat liqueur and brandy, but do not boil. Arrange crêpes around edge of skillet. Pour liqueur into center of skillet and ignite. Spoon flaming sauce over crêpes.

1 serving (total recipe) = 450 calories
                          6 gm protein

# CREPES

1½ cups all-purpose flour
1 tablespoon sugar
¼ teaspoon baking powder
½ teaspoon salt
2 cups milk

2 eggs
½ teaspoon vanilla
2 tablespoons margarine or butter,
  melted

Measure flour, sugar, baking powder, and salt into bowl. Stir in milk, eggs, vanilla, and margarine; beat with rotary beater until smooth.

For each crêpe, lightly grease 8-inch skillet with margarine; heat over medium heat until margarine is bubbly. Pour scant ¼ cup of batter into skillet; immediately rotate pan until batter covers bottom. Cook until light brown on other side. Stack crêpes, placing waxed paper or paper towels between them. Keep crêpes covered to prevent them from drying out.

Use crêpes at once or cool completely, wrap in aluminum foil, and place in freezer. Frozen crêpes will keep for several weeks.

12 to 16 crepes     1 crêpe = 85 calories
                          3 gm protein


# CHOCOLATE MOUSSE PIE

1 package (11½ ounces) milk chocolate pieces
16 large marshmallows
⅛ teaspoon salt

½ cup milk
1 cup chilled whipping cream
8-inch graham cracker crust

Melt chocolate pieces and marshmallows in salt and milk in top of double boiler over hot water. Blend and remove from heat. Cool 1½ hours.

Beat cream in chilled bowl until stiff. Fold into chocolate mixture. Pour into crust. Refrigerate at least 2 hours.

6 servings     ⅙ pie = 755 calories
                      9 gm protein

# PECAN PIE

Pastry for 9-inch one-crust pie
3 eggs
1 cup corn syrup
1 cup sugar

2 tablespoons margarine or butter,
   melted
1 teaspoon vanilla
$\frac{1}{8}$ teaspoon salt
1 cup pecans

Heat oven to 350°. Prepare pastry. Beat eggs slightly in small mixer bowl. Beat in syrup, sugar, margarine, vanilla, and salt. Stir in nuts. Pour into pastry-lined pie pan. Bake 55 to 65 minutes or until knife inserted halfway between center and edge comes out clean. Cool. Nice served with whipped cream.

6 to 8 servings      $\frac{1}{7}$ pie = 455 calories
                          5 gm protein


# STRAWBERRY-YOGURT REFRIGERATOR PIE

*Dessert with a tang for those who don't want a sweet taste.*

2 packages (8 ounces each) cream
   cheese, softened
$\frac{1}{3}$ cup honey
$\frac{1}{4}$ teaspoon salt
1 teaspoon vanilla

1 cup plain yogurt
9-inch graham cracker crust
2 cups sweetened sliced
   strawberries

Beat cream cheese, honey, salt, and vanilla in small mixer bowl until smooth. Beat in yogurt. Pour into crust. Refrigerate 12 hours. Serve with strawberries.

6 to 8 servings      $\frac{1}{7}$ pie = 600 calories
                          10 gm protein

# APPLESAUCE CAKE

2 cups all-purpose flour
1 teaspoon baking soda
¾ teaspoon salt
⅛ teaspoon cloves
1 teaspoon cinnamon
⅓ cup shortening

1 cup brown sugar (packed)
1 egg
1 cup applesauce
1½ teaspoons grated lemon peel
3 tablespoons vinegar
1 cup seedless raisins

Heat oven to 350°. Grease and flour baking pan 8 x 8 x 2 inches. Measure all ingredients except raisins into large mixer bowl. Blend ½ minute at low speed, scraping bowl constantly. Beat 3 minutes at high speed, scraping bowl occasionally. Stir in raisins. Pour into pan.

Bake 35 minutes or until wooden pick inserted in center comes out clean. Superb with whipped cream.

8 servings     1 square = 365 calories
                    4 gm protein

# BOURBON POUND CAKE

8 eggs, separated
3 cups sugar
2 cups margarine or butter, softened (1 pound)
1 tablespoon plus 1 teaspoon vanilla

3 cups all-purpose flour
¼ cup bourbon
1 cup dairy sour cream
1 cup finely chopped pecans
Powdered sugar

Heat oven to 350°. Grease tube pan 10 x 4 inches. Beat egg whites in medium bowl with electric mixer until frothy. Beat in 1 cup of the sugar, 1 tablespoon at a time, until firm peaks are formed. Set aside.

Beat margarine and remaining sugar in large mixer bowl until light and fluffy. Add egg yolks, one at a time, beating after each addition. Mix in vanilla. At low speed, blend in flour alternately with bourbon, scraping bowl frequently. Beat in sour cream until smooth. Fold in meringue with rubber spatula. Stir in pecans. Turn into pan. Bake on lower shelf of oven 1½ hours, until top springs back when touched with finger. (If cake browns too quickly, cover top with aluminum foil.) Remove from oven; cool on wire rack 15 minutes.

Loosen cake around edge; turn onto wire rack and cool completely. At serving time, sprinkle cake with powdered sugar.

16 servings          1 slice = 550 calories
                              7 gm protein

# RUM CAKE

1 cup chopped pecans
1 package (18½ ounces) golden yellow cake mix
1 package (3¾ ounces) instant pudding and pie filling

4 eggs
½ cup water
½ cup vegetable oil
½ cup dark rum
Glaze (below)

Heat oven to 325°. Grease and flour 10-inch tube pan or 12-cup bundt pan. Sprinkle nuts in pan. Empty cake mix into large mixer bowl; add remaining ingredients except glaze. Mix at low speed ½ minute, scraping bowl constantly. Beat at high speed, scraping bowl frequently, until mixture is smooth. Pour into pan. Bake 60 minutes, until cake springs back when touched lightly with finger. Cool in pan.

Invert cake onto large serving plate. Prick top of cake with wooden pick. Drizzle glaze evenly over top and side of cake. Pause to allow cake to absorb glaze. Repeat process until all glaze is used.

*Glaze*
½ cup margarine or butter
¼ cup water

1¼ cups sugar
3 tablespoons dark rum

Melt margarine in small saucepan. Stir in water and sugar; heat to boiling and boil 5 minutes, stirring constantly. Remove from heat; stir in rum.

16 slices          1 slice = 490 calories
                              4 gm protein

NOTE: Cake can be decorated with border of whipped cream and served with small bunches of seedless green grapes dusted with powdered sugar.

# LEMON POUND CAKE

*A very tart but high-calorie delight.*

½ cup butter, softened
1 cup sugar
2 eggs
1 tablespoon lemon juice
½ teaspoon salt

1½ cups all-purpose flour
1 teaspoon baking powder
½ cup milk
⅓ cup lemon juice
¼ cup sugar

Heat oven to 325°. Grease loaf pan 9 x 5 x 3 inches. Cream butter and 1 cup sugar in large mixer bowl until light and fluffy. Beat in eggs and 1 tablespoon lemon juice until smooth. Mix in salt, flour, and baking powder alternately with milk, beating after each addition until batter is smooth. Pour into pan.

Bake 1 hour or until wooden pick inserted in center comes out clean. Mix ⅓ cup lemon juice and ¼ cup sugar. Make holes in top of hot cake with wooden pick. Drizzle lemon-sugar mixture over top of cake. Serve cake warm.

10 slices      1 slice = 300 calories
                        4 gm protein

# CARROT CAKE

2 cups all-purpose flour
2 teaspoons soda
3 teaspoons cinnamon
¾ teaspoon salt
2 cups sugar

4 cups shredded carrot
½ cup vegetable oil
4 eggs
1 cup chopped nuts
Icing (below)

Heat oven to 325°. Grease and flour baking pan 13 x 9 x 2 inches. Measure all ingredients except nuts and icing into large mixer bowl. Blend at low speed ½ minute, scraping bowl constantly. Beat at high speed 3 minutes, scraping bowl frequently. Stir in nuts. Pour into pan.

Bake 40 to 50 minutes or until cake springs back when touched with finger. Cool. Frost with icing.

*Icing*
¼ cup plus 2 tablespoons margarine or butter softened (¾ stick)
1 package (8 ounces) cream cheese, softened
2 cups powdered sugar

1 teaspoon vanilla
Beat margarine and cream cheese in small mixer bowl until fluffy. Add sugar and vanilla; beat until smooth.

15 squares     1 square = 460 calories
                          6 gm protein

NOTE: Substitute 1 cup whole wheat flour for 1 cup of the all-purpose flour.


# GINGERBREAD

2½ cups all-purpose flour
2 teaspoons baking powder
½ teaspoon baking soda
1 teaspoon ginger
1 teaspoon salt
2 teaspoons cinnamon

½ teaspoon cloves
½ cup sugar
½ cup shortening
1 cup dark molasses
2 eggs
1 cup hot water

Heat oven to 350°. Grease baking pan 9 x 9 x 2 inches. Measure all ingredients into large mixer bowl. Blend ½ minute at low speed, scraping bowl constantly. Beat 3 minutes at medium speed, scraping bowl occasionally. Pour into pan.

Bake about 50 minutes or until wooden pick inserted in center comes out clean.

9 servings     1 square = 360 calories
                          5 gm protein

NOTE: Serve with a generous topping of whipped cream or ice cream.

# PASTRY FOR 8 OR 9-INCH ONE-CRUST PIE

1 **cup** all-purpose flour                    2 to 3 tablespoons cold water
⅓ cup plus 1 tablespoon shortening

Measure flour into bowl. Cut in shortening thoroughly. Sprinkle in water, 1 tablespoon at a time, mixing until all flour is moistened, and dough almost cleans side of bowl (1 to 2 tablespoons water can be added if needed).

Gather dough into ball; shape into flattened round on lightly floured cloth-covered board. With floured stockinet-covered rolling pin, roll dough 2 inches larger than inverted pie pan. Fold pastry into quarters; place in pan, unfold, and ease into place. Trim overhanging edge of pastry 1 inch from rim of pan. Fold and roll pastry under, even with pan; flute edges. Fill and bake as directed in recipe.

» *For Baked Pie Shell:* Prick bottom and side thoroughly with fork. Bake at 475° for 8 to 10 minutes.

⅛ pie shell = 140 calories
            1½ gm protein

# *18*

## *DESSERT SAUCES*

## *AND TOPPINGS*

WHIPPED BRANDY CREAM · CHANTILLY CREAM · FRUIT
SYRUPS · HARD SAUCE · RUM SAUCE · SHERRY OR PORT
WINE SAUCE · PUNCHY RUM SAUCE · BLENDER SAUCE
MELBA · FRUIT SUNDAE SAUCE · BRANDY ORANGE SAUCE ·
COFFEE CHOCOLATE SAUCE · CHOCOLATE SAUCE

# WHIPPED BRANDY CREAM

½ cup chilled whipping cream          Grated peel of ½ lemon
1 tablespoon sugar                    2 tablespoons brandy

Beat cream, sugar, and lemon peel in chilled bowl until almost stiff.
Beat in brandy gradually; continue beating until mixture is stiff.
Serve immediately on fruit desserts or hot puddings.

4 servings          ¼ cup = 120 calories
                              1 gm protein

# CHANTILLY CREAM

½ cup chilled whipping cream          1 teaspoon vanilla
¼ cup confectioners' sugar

Beat cream and sugar in chilled bowl until stiff. Fold in vanilla.

2 servings          ½ cup = 240 calories
                              1 gm protein

# FRUIT SYRUPS

*A wonderful topping for pancakes, French toast, waffles, or ice cream.*

» *Strawberry:* Measure 1½ cups sliced strawberries and 1 cup light
corn syrup into blender container. Blend on high speed until
smooth, about 10 seconds. Cover and refrigerate.

2 cups

» *Apricot:* Cook ⅓ cup (packed) dried apricots and 1 cup water in
covered saucepan until apricots are tender and water is absorbed,
10 to 15 minutes. Measure 1 cup light corn syrup into blender container. Add apricots and blend at high speed until smooth. Cover
and refrigerate.

1⅔ cups

» *Pineapple:* Empty 1 can (8 ounces) crushed pineapple in unsweetened pineapple juice and 1 cup light corn syrup into blender container. Blend at high speed until smooth, about 10 seconds. Cover
and refrigerate.

1¾ cups

» *Blackberry:* Place 1 package (10 ounces) frozen blackberries, partially thawed, and 1 cup light corn syrup in blender container. Blend at high speed until smooth, about 10 seconds, or mash berries and corn syrup in bowl with fork until fairly smooth.

2 cups

» *Raspberry:* Substitute 1 package (10 ounces) frozen raspberries, partially thawed, for the blackberries.

» *Peach:* Substitute 1 package (10 ounces) frozen peach slices, partially thawed, for the blackberries.

» *Cherry:* Substitute 1 package (10 ounces) frozen cherries, partially thawed, for the blackberries.

2 tablespoons = approximately 75 calories
              0 protein

NOTE: One and a half cups sliced fresh fruit or berries can be substituted for the frozen fruit.

# HARD SAUCE

$\frac{1}{4}$ cup margarine or butter, softened     $\frac{1}{2}$ teaspoon lemon juice
$\frac{2}{3}$ cup confectioners' sugar          $\frac{1}{2}$ teaspoon vanilla or brandy

Mix all ingredients thoroughly. Cover and refrigerate at least 1 hour. Serve on hot puddings.

About $\frac{1}{3}$ cup      1 tablespoon = 150 calories
                              0 protein

# RUM SAUCE

3 tablespoons sugar             2 tablespoons water
1$\frac{1}{2}$ teaspoons lemon juice     2 tablespoons rum

In small saucepan, heat sugar, lemon juice, and water to boiling, stirring until sugar is dissolved. Cool. Stir in rum. Serve on cake, ice cream, or fruit.

About $\frac{1}{3}$ cup      $\frac{1}{3}$ cup = 216 calories
                              0 protein

## SHERRY OR PORT WINE SAUCE

1 cup margarine or butter, softened  
2 tablespoons sugar  

$\frac{1}{2}$ cup sherry or port  
$1\frac{1}{2}$ ounces brandy  

Beat margarine and sugar in small mixer bowl until fluffy. Heat sherry just to simmering. Pour sherry and brandy gradually into margarine, beating constantly at medium speed. Serve on puddings, ice cream, chilled melon balls, or pineapple chunks.

About $1\frac{1}{2}$ cups     $\frac{1}{4}$ cup = 300 calories  
                            0 protein

## PUNCHY RUM SAUCE

1 cup margarine or butter, softened  
$\frac{1}{2}$ cup sherry  
2 ounces brandy  

$\frac{1}{4}$ cup rum  
Grated peel and juice of $\frac{1}{2}$ lemon  
$\frac{1}{4}$ cup sugar  

Measure all ingredients into top of double boiler. Heat over hot water, beating with rotary beater until mixture is smooth. Serve hot on pudding, ice cream, or fruit.

About $1\frac{3}{4}$ cups     $\frac{1}{4}$ cup = 130 calories  
                            0 protein

## BLENDER SAUCE MELBA

1 package (10 ounces) frozen raspberries, thawed  

$\frac{1}{4}$ cup confectioners' sugar  
$\frac{1}{2}$ teaspoon vanilla  

Place all ingredients in blender; cover and blend at high speed about 30 seconds. Serve on ice cream, sherbet or fruits. If desired, pour sauce into 8″ or 9″ square baking or bread pan, and freeze until firm.

About $1\frac{1}{3}$ cups     $\frac{1}{3}$ cup = 100 calories  
                            $\frac{1}{2}$ gm protein

# FRUIT SUNDAE SAUCE

*Use as a topping for fruit or ice cream.*

2 teaspoons cornstarch
2 teaspoons water
1 cup crushed pineapple

2 tablespoons honey
$\frac{1}{2}$ teaspoon lemon juice

Mix cornstarch and water in small saucepan. Stir in pineapple. Cook, stirring constantly, until mixture thickens and boils. Remove from heat; stir in honey and lemon juice. Cover and refrigerate at least 1 hour.

1 cup        $\frac{1}{4}$ cup = 70 calories
                      0 protein


# BRANDY ORANGE SAUCE

$\frac{1}{2}$ cup margarine, softened
$\frac{1}{2}$ cup confectioners' sugar
$\frac{1}{2}$ cup brandy

2 tablespoons grated orange peel
3 tablespoons orange juice

Mix all ingredients thoroughly. Cover and refrigerate at least 1 hour. Serve on warm apple pie, hot applesauce, or pound cake.

About $\frac{3}{4}$ cup        2 tablespoons = 230 calories
                                    0 protein


# COFFEE CHOCOLATE SAUCE

*Use on ice cream or pound cake.*

2 bars (4 ounces each) sweet cook-
    ing chocolate

1 cup medium-strength coffee

Heat chocolate and coffee over medium heat, stirring constantly, until chocolate is melted, and mixture is smooth.

About 1 cup        $\frac{1}{4}$ cup = 145 calories
                            3 gm protein

# CHOCOLATE SAUCE

2 bars (4 ounces each) sweet cook-        1 cup water
   ing chocolate

Heat chocolate and water over medium heat, stirring constantly,
until chocolate is melted and mixture is smooth. Stir in 1 teaspoon
vanilla if desired.

About 1 cup        $\frac{1}{4}$ cup = 145 calories
                              3 gm protein

# APPENDIX

## Appendix A

### CLEAR LIQUID DIET*

A clear liquid diet includes only foods that are clear and liquid or which liquefy at room temperature—fat-free broth, bouillon, coffee, tea, decaffeinated coffee, strained fruit juices, flavored gelatin, carbonated beverages, and popsicles.

The diet is restrictive and has little nutritive value. It provides some electrolytes, primarily sodium chloride and potassium, and a small amount of kilocalories, mainly in the form of carbohydrates. It is prescribed to supply an oral source of fluids and minimal kilocalories and electrolytes, as a means of preventing dehydration and reducing colonic residue.

This diet should not be used on a long-term basis as the sole means of nutritional support.

If a restricted-sodium clear liquid diet is required, salt-free broth should be substituted for bouillon. Following gastric surgery or myocardial infarction, it may be desirable to eliminate caffeine-containing beverages like coffee, tea, and colas.

SAMPLE MENU

*Morning*
4 oz apple juice
1 cup flavored gelatin
8 oz ginger ale
Coffee or tea with sugar

*Between meals*
$\frac{1}{2}$ cup flavored gelatin

*Noon*
1 cup bouillon
4 oz strained orange juice

$\frac{1}{2}$ cup flavored gelatin
Coffee or tea with sugar

*Between meals*
8 oz ginger ale

*Evening*
1 cup bouillon
4 oz sweetened cranberry juice
$\frac{1}{2}$ cup flavored gelatin
Coffee or tea with sugar

*Bedtime*
$\frac{1}{2}$ cup flavored gelatin

*Adapted from: *Handbook of Clinical Dietetics*, The American Dietetic Association, Yale University Press, New Haven, 1981.

# Appendix B

## MODERATELY RESTRICTED SODIUM DIET*
### (2400–4500 mg Sodium)

1. Do not use salt at the table, and use it sparingly in cooking.
2. Use baking powder, baking soda, or cream of tartar only for baking.
3. Eliminate the following foods:

Salty or smoked meat, such as bacon, bologna, chipped beef, corned beef, frankfurters, ham, meats koshered by salting, luncheon meats, salt pork, sausage, smoked tongue.

Salty or smoked fish, anchovies, caviar, salted cod, herring, sardines, and so on.

Processed cheese or cheese spreads, unless they are low-sodium dietetic products.

Natural, aged cheeses such as Roquefort, Camembert, or Gorgonzola

Regular peanut butter

Sauerkraut, pickles, or other vegetables prepared in brine or heavily salted

Breads and rolls with salt toppings

Salted popcorn

Potato chips, corn chips, crackers and similar salty snacks

Pretzels

Salted nuts

Party spreads and dips

Canned soups, stews, and any kind of commercial bouillon

Instant cocoa mixes

Cooking wine

Olives

Pickles and relishes

Celery salt, garlic salt, onion salt

Catsup and chili sauce

Commercial seasonings made of meat and vegetable extracts

Barbecue sauces and meat sauces

Meat tenderizers

Soy sauce

Worcestershire sauce

*Adapted from: *Handbook of Clinical Dietetics,* The American Dietetic Association, Yale University Press, New Haven, 1981.

# Appendix C

## Foods allowed

**Beverages and Dairy Products**
Carbonated drinks, coffee, freeze-dried coffee, fruit drinks, some instant coffees (check labels), lactose-free milk or milk treated with lactase enzymes; lactose-free dairy products.

**Breads and cereal products**
Breads and rolls made without milk, Italian bread, some cooked cereals and prepared cereals (read labels), macaroni, spaghetti, soda crackers.

**Desserts**
Water and fruit ices; gelatin; angel food cake; homemade cakes, pies, cookies, made from allowed ingredients; puddings made with water.

**Eggs**

**Fats**
Margarines and dressings that do not contain milk or milk products; oils, shortening; bacon;

## Foods excluded

**Beverages and Dairy Products**
All untreated milk—skim, dried, evaporated, or condensed—and all products containing untreated milk: yogurt; cheese; ice cream; sherbet; malted milk; Ovaltine; hot chocolate; some cocoas and instant coffees (read labels); powdered soft drinks with lactose curds; milk that has been treated with lactobacillus/acidophilus culture rather than lactase.

**Breads and cereal products**
Prepared mixes for muffins, biscuits, waffles, pancakes; some dry cereals (read labels); instant cream of wheat; commercial breads and rolls to which milk solids have been added; zwieback; French toast made with milk.

**Desserts**
Commercial cakes, cookies, and mixes; custard, puddings, sherbets, or ice cream made with milk; products containing chocolate; pie crust made with butter or margarine; gelatin made with carrageen.

**Eggs**
Omelets, quiches, and soufflés containing milk, cheese, chocolate or other untreated dairy products.

**Fats**
Margarines and dressings containing milk or milk products; butter, cream; cream cheese; peanut

*Adapted from: *Handbook of Clinical Dietetics*, The American Dietetic Association, Yale University Press, New Haven, 1981.

| Foods allowed | Foods excluded |
|---|---|
| some whipped toppings and some nondairy creamers (read labels); nut butters and nuts. | butter with milk-solids fillers; salad dressings containing lactose. |
| *Fruits* | *Fruits* |
| All fresh, canned, or frozen fruits not processed with lactose. | Any canned or frozen fruits processed with lactose. |
| *Meat, fish, poultry* | *Meat, fish, poultry* |
| Plain beef, chicken, fish, turkey, lamb, veal, pork, and ham; strained or junior meats and vegetables and meat combinations that do not contain milk or milk products; kosher frankfurters. | Creamed or breaded meat, fish, or fowl; sausage products such as frankfurters, liver sausage, or cold cuts that contain nonfat milk solids. |
| *Soups* | *Soups* |
| Clear soups, vegetable soups, consommés, cream soups made with nondairy creamers. | Cream soups, except for those made with allowed ingredients; chowders; commercially prepared soups containing lactose. |
| *Vegetables* | *Vegetables* |
| Fresh, canned, or frozen artichokes, asparagus, broccoli, cabbage, carrots, cauliflower, celery, chard, corn, cucumber, eggplant, green beans, kale, lettuce, mustard, okra, onions, parsley, parsnips, pumpkin, rutabaga, spinach, squash, tomatoes, white and sweet potatoes, yams, lima beans, beets. | Any to which lactose is added during processing; peas; creamed, breaded, or buttered vegetables; instant potatoes; corn curls; frozen French fries processed with lactose. |
| *Miscellaneous* | *Miscellaneous* |
| Soy sauce, carob powder, popcorn, olives, sugar, pure sugar candy, jelly or marmalade, corn syrup, carbonated beverages, gravy made with water, Baker's cocoa, pickles, pure seasonings and spices, wine, molasses (beet sugar), pure monosodium glutamate, instant coffees that do not contain lactose. | Chewing gum; most chocolate; some cocoa; toffee; peppermint; butterscotch; caramels; some instant coffees; some dietetic preparations (read labels); some antibiotics and vitamin and mineral preparations; spice blends containing milk products; monosodium glutamate extenders; artificial sweeteners containing lactose; some nondairy creamers (read labels). |

# Appendix D

## FAT-RESTRICTED DIET*
### (50 grams)

| *Foods allowed* | *Foods excluded* |
|---|---|
| **Beverages** | **Beverages** |
| Skim milk or buttermilk made with skim milk; coffee, tea, Postum; fruit juice; soft drinks; cocoa made with cocoa powder and skim milk. | Whole milk, buttermilk made with whole milk, chocolate milk, cream in excess of the fat allowance in the diet. |
| **Bread and cereal products** | **Bread and cereal products** |
| Plain, nonfat cereals; spaghetti, noodles, rice, macaroni; plain whole-grain or enriched bread. | Muffins, biscuits, breads, egg or cheese bread; sweet rolls made with fat; pancakes, doughnuts, waffles, fritters; popcorn prepared with fat; natural cereals and breads to which extra fat is added. |
| **Cheese** | **Cheese** |
| Low-fat cottage cheese or specially processed American cheese containing less than 5% butterfat. | Whole milk cheeses. |
| **Desserts** | **Desserts** |
| Sherbet made with skim milk; fruit ice; gelatin; rice, bread, cornstarch, tapioca, or Junket puddings made with skim milk; fruit whips with gelatin, sugar, and egg white; fruit; angel food cake; meringues. | Cake, pie, pastry, ice cream—all desserts containing shortening, chocolate, or fats of any kind, unless the fat contained is within the daily fat allowance. |
| **Eggs** | **Eggs** |
| 3 per week, prepared only with fat from the fat allowance; egg whites as desired; low-fat egg substitutes. | More than 3 a week unless substituted for part of the meat allowance. |

*Adapted from: *Handbook of Clinical Dietetics*, The American Dietetic Association, Yale University Press, New Haven, 1981.

| Foods allowed | Foods excluded |
|---|---|

**Fats**

Choose up to 5 or 6 servings from the following (1 serving in the amount listed equals 1 fat choice):

1 tsp butter of fortified margarine
1 tsp shortening or oil
1 tsp mayonnaise
1 tbsp Italian or French dressing
1 strip crisp bacon
⅛ avocado (4" diameter)
2 tbsp light cream
1 tbsp heavy cream
6 small nuts
5 small olives

**Fats**

Any in excess of amount prescribed.

**Fruits**

As desired.

**Fruits**

Avocado in excess of amount allowed on fat list.

**Meat, fish, poultry**

Choose up to 6 ounces from the following: poultry without skin; fish; veal (all cuts); liver; lean beef, pork, and lamb with all visible fat removed (1 ounce cooked weight equals 1 equivalent); ¼ cup water-packed tuna or salmon equals 1 ounce of meat.

**Meat, fish, poultry**

Fried or fatty meats; sausage, scrapple, frankfurters, poultry skin, stewing hens, spareribs, salt pork, beef that is not lean, duck, goose, ham hocks, pigs' feet, luncheon meats, gravies (unless fat free), tuna and salmon packed in oil, peanut butter.

**Milk**

Skim milk or buttermilk or yogurt made from skim mulk.

**Milk**

Whole or chocolate milk or buttermilk made from whole milk.

**Seasonings**

As desired.

**Seasonings**

As desired.

**Soups**

Bouillon, clear broth, fat-free vegetable soup, cream soup made with skimmed milk, packaged dehydrated soups.

**Soups**

All others are prohibited.

**Sweets**

Jelly, jam, marmalade, honey, syrup, molasses, sugar, hard sugar candies, fondant, gumdrops, jelly beans, marshmallows.

**Sweets**

Any candy made with chocolate, nuts, butter, cream, or fat of any kind.

| Food allowed | Foods excluded |
|---|---|
| *Vegetables* | *Vegetables* |
| All vegetables prepared without fats. | Potato chips; buttered, au gratin, creamed, or fried vegetables unless the fat contained is within the daily fat allowance; commercially frozen vegetables or casseroles, or frozen vegetables in butter sauce. |

# Appendix E

### DIETARY FIBER CONTENT OF SELECTED FOODS*

Estimated daily adult requirement of crude fiber/day is 6 gm

| Fruits | Portion Sizes | Total Dietary Fiber (gm)/Serving |
|---|---|---|
| Apples | 1 med | 2.41 |
| Bananas | one 6 in | 1.75 |
| Cherries | 25 sm/med | 1.24 |
| Guavas (canned) | 1 med | 3.62 |
| Peaches | 1 med | 2.28 |
| Pears | $\frac{1}{2}$ med | 2.07 |
| Plums | 2 med | 1.52 |
| Rhubarb (raw) | $\frac{1}{2}$ cup | 1.07 |
| Strawberries (raw) | 10 lg | 2.12 |
| *Nuts* | | |
| Brazil | $\frac{1}{4}$ cup | 2.71 |
| *Peanut Butter* | 1 tbsp | 1.13 |
| *Leafy Vegetables* | | |
| Broccoli tops (boiled) | $\frac{1}{2}$ cup | 2.99 |
| Brussels sprouts | $\frac{1}{2}$ cup | 2.00 |
| Cabbage | $\frac{1}{2}$ cup | 2.07 |
| Cauliflower | $\frac{1}{2}$ cup | 1.13 |
| Onions (raw) | one $2\frac{1}{4}$ in | 2.10 |
| *Legumes* | | |
| Beans (baked) | $\frac{1}{3}$ cup | 6.18 |
| Peas, frozen | $\frac{1}{2}$ cup | 5.66 |

*Adapted from: *Handbook of Clinical Dietetics,* The American Dietetic Association, Yale University Press, New Haven, 1981.

| Root Vegetables | Portion Sizes | Total Dietary Fiber (gm)/Serving |
|---|---|---|
| Carrots, young (boiled) | $\frac{1}{2}$ cup | 2.78 |
| Parsnips (raw) | $\frac{1}{2}$ lg | 4.90 |
| Potato, Maine (raw) | one $2\frac{1}{4}$ in | 3.51 |
| Tomatoes (fresh) | 1 sm | 1.40 |
| Sweet corn, cooked | $\frac{1}{2}$ ear | 2.37 |
| *Flours* | | |
| Whole grain | $\frac{1}{2}$ cup | 6.28 |
| Bran | $\frac{1}{2}$ cup | 13.20 |
| Whole grain bread | 1 slice | 1.96 |
| *Breakfast Cereals* | | |
| All Bran | $\frac{3}{4}$ cup | 11.20 |
| Grape-Nuts | $\frac{3}{4}$ cup | 5.88 |
| Shredded wheat | 1 biscuit | 2.70 |

*Examples of High and Low Fiber Foods*

2 slices whole grain bread contains 3.14 gm total dietary fiber
2 slices white bread contains 0.71 gm total dietary fiber

All bran cereal contains 7.6 gm total dietary fiber/oz
Rice Krispies contains 1.28 gm total dietary fiber/oz

$\frac{1}{2}$ cup lima beans contains 3.16 gm total dietary fiber
$\frac{1}{2}$ cup cauliflower contains 1.13 gm total dietary fiber

$\frac{1}{2}$ ear sweet corn contains 2.37 gm total dietary fiber
$\frac{1}{2}$ cup summer squash contains 0.37 gm total dietary fiber

1 medium pear contains 4.14 gm total dietary fiber
1 orange contains 0.65 gm total dietary fiber

# Appendix F

## FIBER-RESTRICTED DIET*

A low-fiber diet is not necessarily a low-residue diet because some low-fiber foods increase stool weight by other mechanisms. Prune juice, for example, increases colonic residue by its laxative action.

To adapt this low-fiber diet to a low-residue regimen, restrict the fruits and vegetables in the diet to strained fruit and vegetable juices and white potatoes without skin. All other forms should be eliminated.

*Adapted from: *Handbook of Clinical Dietetics*, The American Dietetic Association, Yale University Press, New Haven, 1981.

In addition, milk may indirectly contribute to fecal residue, although it contains no crude fiber, so it may be wise to limit milk intake to 2 cups a day.

| *Foods allowed* | *Foods excluded* |
|---|---|
| *Beverages* | *Beverages* |
| Milk, carbonated beverages, Postum, cider, coffee, tea. | Drinks made from prohibited vegetables and fruits or other foods not allowed. |
| *Bread and cereal products* | *Bread and cereal products* |
| White bread and toast; melba toast; crackers; bagels; cereals; waffles; French toast; refined cereals such as cream of wheat, cream of rice, cornflakes, puffed rice. | Coarse whole-grain breads and cereals, especially bran flakes, cracked wheat, Grape-Nuts, Grape-Nuts Flakes. |
| *Desserts* | *Desserts* |
| Plain cakes and cookies; gelatin; plain puddings; custard; any plain desserts made from allowed foods without nuts, raisins, fruits, or coconut, e.g., ice cream, ices, Popsicles. | Coconut, raisins, fruits, nuts, or any desserts made with other foods not allowed. |
| *Fats* | *Fats* |
| Butter, margarine, salad oils, mayonnaise, cream, crisp bacon, plain gravies, plain salad dressings. | Nuts, olives. |
| *Fruits* | *Fruits* |
| Strained fruit juices, except prune, and canned fruit, except those on the excluded list. | Any not allowed, especially dates, figs, prunes, boysenberries, blackberries, blueberries, kumquats, pineapple, rhubarb, avocados, grapes, apples, peaches, pears, guavas, fresh grapefruit and orange sections. |
| *Meat and meat substitutes* | *Meat and meat substitutes* |
| Ground or well-cooked, tender beef, ham, veal, lamb, pork, poultry, steak and chops, fish, oysters, shrimp, lobster, clams, liver, crab, organ meats, eggs, cheese. | Tough, fibrous meats with gristle; peanut butter, smooth or chunky. |
| *Soups and miscellaneous* | *Soups and miscellaneous* |
| Strained soups made from allowed foods; arrowroot; candy, such as butterscotch, jelly beans, marsh- | Chocolate nut bars or peanut brittle, pickles, sesame seed, any soup made from vegetables not |

| Foods allowed | Foods excluded |
|---|---|
| mallows, plain hard candy; cornstarch; gelatin; honey, molasses, sugar; catsup, vinegar, prepared mustard; and the following spices, which contain less than 0.015 g fiber per $\frac{1}{8}$ tsp: | on allowed lists; and any other foods not on allowed lists. |

Allspice
Basil
Bay leaves
Celery salt, powder, or leaves
Cinnamon
Cumin powder
Ginger
Mace
Marjoram
Onion powder
Oregano
Paprika
Parsley flakes
Pepper, black, ground
Rosemary
Sage
Savory
Tarragon
Thyme
Turmeric

*Vegetables*
Strained vegetables and their juice; lettuce; cooked asparagus, beets, green beans, tomatoes; eggplant; acorn squash without seeds; lima beans; spinach.

*Vegetables*
Any not allowed, especially peas, parsnips, rutabaga, broccoli, Brussels sprouts, cabbage, onions, carrots, turnips, cauliflower, baked beans, fresh tomatoes, zucchini, corn.

# Appendix G

## MANUFACTURERS OF LIQUID FORMULAS

| Company | Product |
|---|---|
| Beecham-Massengill Pharmaceuticals Melrose, MA 02176 | Hy/cal (supplement) |
| Biosearch Medical Products, Inc. 35 Industrial Parkway P.O. Box 1700 Somerville, NJ 08876 | Magnacal (complete nutritional feeding) Microlipid (supplement) Renu (complete nutritional feeding) Sumacal (supplement) Vitaneed (complete nutritional feeding) |

| Company | Product |
|---|---|
| Carnation Company<br>Los Angeles, CA 90036 | Carnation Instant Breakfast (complete nutritional feeding) |
| Delmark Food Service Company<br>Minneapolis, MN 55416 | High Protein Gelatin Mix (supplement) |
| Doyle Pharmaceutical Company<br>5320 West 23 Street<br>Minneapolis, MN 55416 | Citrotein (supplement)<br>Compleat B (complete nutritional feeding)<br>Compleat-Modified (complete nutritional feeding)<br>Isotein HN<br>Meritene (complete nutritional feeding)<br>Precision HN (complete nutritional feeding)<br>Precision Isotonic (complete nutritional feeding)<br>Precision LR (complete nutritional feeding) |
| Henkel Corporation<br>4620 West 77th Street<br>Minneapolis, MN 55435 | Cal-Plus (supplement) |
| Lederle Laboratories<br>Division American Cyanamid<br>Company<br>Pearl River, NY 10965 | Gevral Protein (supplement) |
| Mead Johnson<br>Nutritional Division<br>2404 Pennsylvania Avenue<br>Evansville, IN 47721 | Casec (supplement)<br>Criticare (defined-formula feeding)<br>Isocal (complete nutritional feeding)<br>Isocal HCN (complete nutritional feeding)<br>MCT Oil (supplement)<br>Moducal (supplement)<br>Portagen (complete nutritional feeding)<br>Sustacal (complete nutritional feeding)<br>Sustacal HC (complete nutritional feeding)<br>Sustacal Pudding (supplement)<br>Traumacal |
| NAVACO Laboratories<br>Box 23162<br>Phoenix, AZ 85063 | Pro Mix (supplement) |
| Norwich-Eaton Pharmaceuticals<br>17 Eaton Avenue<br>Norwich, NY 13815 | Vivonex (defined-formula feeding)<br>Vivonex HN (defined-formula feeding) |

| Company | Product |
|---|---|
| Ross Laboratories<br>625 Cleveland Avenue<br>Columbus, OH 43216 | Ensure (complete nutritional feeding)<br>Ensure Plus (complete nutritional feeding)<br>Forta Pudding (supplement)<br>Osmolite (complete nutritional feeding)<br>Polycose (supplement)<br>Vital (defined-formula feeding) |
| Travenol Laboratories, Inc.<br>1 Baxter Parkway<br>Deerfield, IL 60015 | Travasorb HN (defined-formula feeding)<br>Travasorb Liquid (complete nutritional feeding)<br>Travasorb MCT (complete nutritional feeding)<br>Travasorb Standard (defined-formula feeding) |

# Appendix H

## COMMERCIALLY AVAILABLE SALIVA SUBSTITUTES

The following saliva substitutes products contain sodium, potassium, and other electrolytes:

| Product | Manufacturer |
|---|---|
| MOI-STIR<br>4 oz bottle with pump and spray<br>  available by direct mail.<br>(317) 846-7452 | Kingswood Laboratories<br>336 Heather Drive<br>P.O. Box 744<br>Carmel, IN 46032 |
| SAL-EZE<br>4 oz bottle or quart refillable<br>  container<br>(800) 426-5913 | North Pacific Dental, Inc.<br>Riverside Business Park<br>15500 N.E. 90th Street<br>Redmond, WA 98052<br>(or)<br>P.O. Box 522<br>Kirkland, WA 98033 |
| SALIV-AID<br>2 oz or 6 oz bottles<br>(617) 268-1208 | Copley Pharmaceuticals<br>398 West Second Street<br>Boston, MA 02127 |
| SALIVART<br>75 gm spray can<br>(203) 226-0622 | Westport Pharmaceuticals<br>P.O. Box 816<br>Westport, CT 06881 |
| SALIVA SUBSTITUTE<br>120 ml squeeze bottle<br>(800) 848-0120<br>(614) 228-5403 | Roxane<br>330 Oak Street<br>Columbus, Ohio 43216 |
| XERO-LUBE<br>6 oz bottle<br>(800) 527-0222 | Scherer Laboratories, Inc.<br>14335 Gillis Road<br>P.O. Drawer 40009<br>Dallas, TX 75240 |

# Appendix I

## BLENDERIZED TUBE FEEDING FORMULA

This formula is based on a normal, well-balanced diet. The proportions have been carefully calculated to supply 2000 calories and adequate protein, minerals, and vitamins.

| *Recipe* | *Equipment Needed* |
|---|---|
| 1 cup farina, cooked, enriched | Blender |
| 3 eggs, cooked | Standard measuring cup |
| 4 tablespoons skim milk powder | Standard measuring spoons |
| 7 ounces ground, lean meat, cooked | Large household mesh strainer |
| $\frac{1}{2}$ cup carrots, canned | Mixing bowl or container, 4-quart capacity |
| $\frac{1}{2}$ cup wax beans, canned | Containers to keep formula in |
| $\frac{1}{4}$ cup corn oil | refrigerator, such as easily |
| $1\frac{1}{2}$ cups orange juice | cleaned quart-size glass bottles |
| $\frac{1}{2}$ cup Karo syrup, dark | or jars (3) each. |
| $\frac{1}{2}$ teaspoon salt | Bottle brush for washing jars |
| 2 cups water and juice from canned vegetables | |
| 1 multi-vitamin tablet | |

## Method of Preparation

1. Make fresh daily.
2. Meat may be lean, ground round of beef, or cooked turkey, chicken or lean cooked beef. If raw beef is used, cook it until it loses its red color. Drain off fat. If cooked meat is used, trim off skin and gristle, cut into cubes.
3. Cook the farina and eggs. The eggs may be scrambled in some of the oil allowance, or stirred into the hot farina.
4. Always start with some liquid in the blender (about 1 cup).
5. Add some solid ingredients, a small amount at a time, until the blender is half full.
6. Blend until smooth.
7. Pour through the strainer into the large container.
8. Repeat in small batches until all the ingredients are used.
9. Vitamin tablet is to be thoroughly crushed with a spoon, added directly to the last batch and blended for a few minutes.

NOTE: In an emergency baby foods may be substituted to meet your requirements. Carnation Instant breakfast is also an acceptable emergency substitute if milk products are tolerated well and will meet your requirements.

Source: Memorial Sloan-Kettering Cancer Center Food Service Department.

10. Add water, if necessary, to make a total quantity of 2000 cc or $2\frac{1}{4}$ qts, enough for one day. This will give five (5) feedings of 400 cc (14 oz.) per feeding.
11. Store the formula in clean containers in the refrigerator.
12. Warm the formula to room temperature or luke warm by setting the portion in a warm water bath before feeding.

# Appendix J

## RECOMMENDED DAILY DIETARY ALLOWANCES

**FOOD AND NUTRITION BOARD, NATIONAL ACADEMY OF SCIENCES—NATIONAL RESEARCH COUNCIL RECOMMENDED DAILY DIETARY ALLOWANCES,[a] REVISED 1980**

Designed for the maintenance of good nutrition of practically all healthy people in the U.S.A.

| | Age (years) | Weight (kg) | Weight (lb) | Height (cm) | Height (in) | Protein (g) | Vita-min A ($\mu$g RE)[b] | Vita-min D ($\mu$g)[c] | Vita-min E (mg $\alpha$-TE)[d] |
|---|---|---|---|---|---|---|---|---|---|
| | | | | | | | Fat-Soluble Vitamins | | |
| Infants | 0.0−0.5 | 6 | 13 | 60 | 24 | kg × 2.2 | 420 | 10 | 3 |
| | 0.5−1.0 | 9 | 20 | 71 | 28 | kg × 2.0 | 400 | 10 | 4 |
| Children | 1–3 | 13 | 29 | 90 | 35 | 23 | 400 | 10 | 5 |
| | 4–6 | 20 | 44 | 112 | 44 | 30 | 500 | 10 | 6 |
| | 7–10 | 28 | 62 | 132 | 52 | 34 | 700 | 10 | 7 |
| Males | 11–14 | 45 | 99 | 157 | 62 | 45 | 1000 | 10 | 8 |
| | 15–18 | 66 | 145 | 176 | 69 | 56 | 1000 | 10 | 10 |
| | 19–22 | 70 | 154 | 177 | 70 | 56 | 1000 | 7.5 | 10 |
| | 23–50 | 70 | 154 | 178 | 70 | 56 | 1000 | 5 | 10 |
| | 51+ | 70 | 154 | 178 | 70 | 56 | 1000 | 5 | 10 |
| Females | 11–14 | 46 | 101 | 157 | 62 | 46 | 800 | 10 | 8 |
| | 15–18 | 55 | 120 | 163 | 64 | 46 | 800 | 10 | 8 |
| | 19–22 | 55 | 120 | 163 | 64 | 44 | 800 | 7.5 | 8 |
| | 23–50 | 55 | 120 | 163 | 64 | 44 | 800 | 5 | 8 |
| | 51+ | 55 | 120 | 163 | 64 | 44 | 800 | 5 | 8 |
| Pregnant | | | | | | +30 | +200 | +5 | +2 |
| Lactating | | | | | | +20 | +400 | +5 | +3 |

[a] The allowances are intended to provide for individual variations among most normal persons as they live in the United States under usual environmental stresses. Diets should be based on a variety of common foods in order to provide other nutrients for which human requirements have been less well defined. See Table 2.2 (p.14) for weights and heights by individual year of age.

[b] Retinol equivalents. 1 retinol equivalent = 1 $\mu$g retinol or 6 $\mu$g $\beta$ carotene. See text for calculation of vitamin A activity of diets as retinol equivalents.

[c] As cholecalciferol. 10 $\mu$g cholecalciferol = 400 IU of vitamin D.

[d] $\alpha$-tocopherol equivalents. 1 mg d-$\alpha$ tocopherol = 1 $\alpha$-TE. See text for variation in allowances and calculation of vitamin E activity of the diet as $\alpha$-tocopherol equivalents.

[e] 1 NE (niacin equivalent) is equal to 1 mg of niacin or 60 mg of dietary tryptophan.

| Water-Soluble Vitamins | | | | | | | Minerals | | | | | |
|---|---|---|---|---|---|---|---|---|---|---|---|---|
| Vita-min C (mg) | Thia-min (mg) | Ribo-flavin (mg) | Niacin (mg NE)[e] | Vita-min B-6 (mg) | Fola-cin[f] (µg) | Vita-min B-12 (µg) | Cal-cium (mg) | Phos-phorus (mg) | Mag-nesium (mg) | Iron (mg) | Zinc (mg) | Iodine (µg) |
| 35 | 0.3 | 0.4 | 6 | 0.3 | 30 | 0.5[g] | 360 | 240 | 50 | 10 | 3 | 40 |
| 35 | 0.5 | 0.6 | 8 | 0.6 | 45 | 1.5 | 540 | 360 | 70 | 15 | 5 | 50 |
| 45 | 0.7 | 0.8 | 9 | 0.9 | 100 | 2.0 | 800 | 800 | 150 | 15 | 10 | 70 |
| 45 | 0.9 | 1.0 | 11 | 1.3 | 200 | 2.5 | 800 | 800 | 200 | 10 | 10 | 90 |
| 45 | 1.2 | 1.4 | 16 | 1.6 | 300 | 3.0 | 800 | 800 | 250 | 10 | 10 | 120 |
| 50 | 1.4 | 1.6 | 18 | 1.8 | 400 | 3.0 | 1200 | 1200 | 350 | 18 | 15 | 150 |
| 60 | 1.4 | 1.7 | 18 | 2.0 | 400 | 3.0 | 1200 | 1200 | 400 | 18 | 15 | 150 |
| 60 | 1.5 | 1.7 | 19 | 2.2 | 400 | 3.0 | 800 | 800 | 350 | 10 | 15 | 150 |
| 60 | 1.4 | 1.6 | 18 | 2.2 | 400 | 3.0 | 800 | 800 | 350 | 10 | 15 | 150 |
| 60 | 1.2 | 1.4 | 16 | 2.2 | 400 | 3.0 | 800 | 800 | 350 | 10 | 15 | 150 |
| 50 | 1.1 | 1.3 | 15 | 1.8 | 400 | 3.0 | 1200 | 1200 | 300 | 18 | 15 | 150 |
| 60 | 1.1 | 1.3 | 14 | 2.0 | 400 | 3.0 | 1200 | 1200 | 300 | 18 | 15 | 150 |
| 60 | 1.1 | 1.3 | 14 | 2.0 | 400 | 3.0 | 800 | 800 | 300 | 18 | 15 | 150 |
| 60 | 1.0 | 1.2 | 13 | 2.0 | 400 | 3.0 | 800 | 800 | 300 | 18 | 15 | 150 |
| 60 | 1.0 | 1.2 | 13 | 2.0 | 400 | 3.0 | 800 | 800 | 300 | 10 | 15 | 150 |
| +20 | +0.4 | +0.3 | +2 | +0.6 | +400 | +1.0 | +400 | +400 | +150 | h | +5 | +25 |
| +40 | +0.5 | +0.5 | +5 | +0.5 | +100 | +1.0 | +400 | +400 | +150 | h | +10 | +50 |

[f]The folacin allowances refer to dietary sources as determined by *Lactobacillus casei* assay after treatment with enzymes (conjugases) to make polyglutamyl forms of the vitamin available to the test organism.

[g]The recommended dietary allowance for vitamin B-12 in infants is based on concentration of the vitamin in human milk. The allowances after weaning are based on energy intake (as recommended by the American Academy of Pediatrics) and consideration of other factors, such as intestinal absorption; see text.

[h]The increased requirement during pregnancy cannot be met by the iron content of habitual American diets nor by the existing iron stores of many women; therefore the use of 30–60 mg of supplemental iron is recommended. Iron needs during lactation are not substantially different from those of nonpregnant women, but continued supplementation of the mother for 2–3 months after parturition is advisable in order to replenish stores depleted by pregnancy.

# GLOSSARY

*Absorption:* The process by which the products of digestion are transferred from the intestinal tract into the blood and lymph circulation.

*Acute:* Occurring suddenly or over a short period of time.

*Amino acids:* Organic compounds of carbon, hydrogen, oxygen, and nitrogen; the building blocks of protein molecules.

*Anorexia:* Lack or loss of appetite for food.

*Bone marrow:* The material which fills the cavities of the bones and is the substance from which the circulating blood cells are formed.

*Cachexia:* A condition which refers to malnutrition and wasting which may occur during the course of an illness.

*Calorie:* A unit of heat measurement: The amount of heat energy needed to raise the temperature of a gram of water one degree centigrade.

*Cancer:* Malignant disease marked by abnormal growth of cells; normal tissues can be invaded by abnormal cells. The abnormal cells can also leave the original site and form new colonies elsewhere in the body.

*Carbohydrate:* A class of substances which includes sugars, starches, and celluloses.

*Cell:* The smallest unit of living material that can function independently.

*Chemotherapy:* The use of chemical agents in treatment of disease.

*Chronic:* A term that is often used to describe a disease of long duration or one that is progressing slowly.

*Colostomy:* A temporary or permanent opening in the abdominal wall to permit elimination of wastes.

*Complete liquid nutritional formula:* Nutrients provided from natural foods or prepared synthetically which will meet normal nutritional requirements if used in adequate amounts; therefore, may be taken as the sole source of nutrition.

*Constipation:* Infrequent or difficult evacuation of the feces.

*Dehydration:* A condition resulting from a loss of water; often results from severe diarrhea.

*Diarrhea:* Frequency of bowel action, soft or liquid stools.

*Diuretics:* Drugs that increase the elimination of water and salt from the body as urine.

*Dumping syndrome:* Body reaction in which food is "dumped" from the stomach into the intestine shortly after being swallowed.

*Dysphagia:* Difficulty in swallowing.

*Edema:* The accumulation of fluid within the tissues.

*Electrolytes:* A general term for the many minerals, particularly sodium and potassium, necessary to provide the proper environment for body cells and proper fluid balance.

*Enzymes:* Complex organic compounds (proteins) produced within an organism which control the rate of chemical reactions in the body.

*Essential fatty acids:* Specific components of dietary fats which are vital to normal metabolism; they cannot be produced by the body and must be obtained from the diet.

*Fat:* Substances such as neutral fats, oils, fatty acids, and cholesterol.

*Food aversion:* A dislike for food in general or a specific type of food.

*Gastrectomy:* Surgical removal of all or part of the stomach.

*Gastrointestinal tract:* The tubular passage that extends from mouth to anus and functions in digestion and absorption of food and elimination of waste. The organs involved in the digestive process, including the esophagus, stomach, intestines, colon, liver, gall bladder, and pancreas. Also referred to as the digestive or alimentary tract.

*Gram:* A metric unit of mass and weight; there are approximately 30 grams in an ounce and 15.432 grains in a gram. Abbreviated g or gm.

*Hormone:* A chemical substance that is produced by the endocrine glands and is carried in body fluids to other organs or parts of the body. Hormones help to regulate the various bodily functions.

*Ileostomy:* Surgical creation of an opening into the ileum usually by establishing an ileal stoma on the abdominal wall.

*Immunotherapy:* A method of cancer therapy which involves stimulating the body's immune defenses.

*Infection:* Refers to the invasion of the body by disease-producing organisms.

*Intravenous (IV):* The administration of a drug or fluid directly into a vein.

*Kilogram:* A metric unit of mass and weight equal to 1000 grams or 2.2046 pounds. Abbreviated kg.

*Lactase:* A specific enzyme found in the small intestine which converts lactose (milk sugar) into glucose and galactose.

*Lactose:* The form of carbohydrate in milk; milk sugar.

*Localized:* Not general; restricted to a limited region or to one or more spots.

*Lymphatic system:* Refers to the lymphoid organs and the circulatory network of vessels that carry lymph fluid.

*Metabolism:* Refers to the physical and chemical changes that occur within a body to provide energy for vital processes and activities.

*Metastasis:* The spread of cancer cells and establishment of new groups of those cells at locations distant from the primary tumor.

*Modality:* A general term for a type of method or treatment. The basic modalities of cancer therapy include surgery, radiotherapy, chemotherapy, and experimental immunotherapy. Multimodality therapy refers to the use of more than one therapy.

*Mucous membrane:* Type of tissue lining body passages open to the outside, such as the gastrointestinal tract.

*Nutrient:* A substance that is necessary for growth, normal functioning, tissue repair, and maintaining life. Essential nutrients are proteins, minerals, fats, carbohydrates, and vitamins.

*Oncology:* The study of physical, chemical, and biological properties and features of cancer.

*Organ:* Several tissues grouped together to perform one or more functions in the body.

*Ostomy:* A suffix which refers to a surgically created passage connecting an internal organ with the skin; see colostomy.

*Queasy:* Uneasy feeling of impending nausea.

*Protein:* Any of numerous, naturally occurring, extremely complex combinations of amino acids that contain the elements carbon, hydrogen, nitrogen, oxygen, etc. and are essential constituents of all living cells.

*Radiation:* The release of energy through waves (such as ultraviolet rays or x-rays) or energetic particles (such as electrons or neutrons).

*Radiotherapy:* A treatment which is based on the capacity of atomic particles and rays to destroy living cells.

*RDA (recommended dietary allowances):* Quantities of specified vitamins, minerals, and protein needed daily for good nutrition.

*Regional:* Pertaining to, limited to, or affecting a certain region or regions.

*Secretion:* A discharge of a substance by a cell or gland.

*Stomatitis:* The inflammation of the mucous membranes in the mouth.

*Syndrome:* A set of symptoms occurring together.

*Tissue:* A collection of cells similar in structure and function.

*Tolerance:* The ability to endure or withstand a particular drug or treatment without ill effects.

*Toxicity:* The quality of a substance which causes ill effects; poisonous.

*TPN:* Total parenteral nutrition; procedure in which nutrients are supplied directly to the bloodstream.

*Trace element:* Chemical elements that are distributed throughout the tissues in very small amounts.

*Tumor:* A mass or swelling; the word "tumor" carries no connotation of being either benign or malignant.

*Vitamin:* Any one of a group of chemical substances vital for the maintenance and growth of the body.

# GENERAL INDEX

Absorption of food, 19
*Acute Lymphoblastic Leukemia (ALL) of Childhood: A Pamphlet for Parents* (Sallan), 58
Adolescents:
    information for, 53
    *see also* Children with cancer
Aker, S., 99
Alcohol, appetite and, 22
Allspice, 65
Alternative therapies, 78–83
American Cancer Society, 56, 87–91, 102–3
    chartered divisions of, 88–91
    on unproven methods of treatment, 79
American Heart Association, 105
American Medical Association, 101
Anesthesiologist, 3
Anesthetic lozenges and sprays, 25
Anise, 65
Anorexia (loss of appetite), 20–22
Anrod, B., 99
Anxiety, appetite and weight loss and, 21
Appetite:
    of children with cancer, 48
    facing an unwanted meal and lack of, 76
    stimulation of, 32–33

Appetite loss, 20–22
    oral cavity surgery and, 40
Aroma, *see* Odor of food
Association for the Study of Childhood Cancer, 58
At-Home Rehabilitation Program of University Hospitals Cancer Center, 52, 57
Aversions to food, 22–23

Bacon, 61
Baker, L. S., 52
Basic four food groups, 11, 12
Basil, 65
Bay leaves, 65
*Bereaved Parent, The* (Schiff), 58
Beverages:
    feeling of fullness and, 26
    loss of appetite and, 22
"Blenderized Diet" (Kukachka), 100
Brody, J. E., 99
Burnet, 65
Butter, 51

Calories (calorie intake), 11
    increasing, 60–61
    estimating requirement for, 13
    snacks high in, 63–64

Cancer:
    definition of, 2
    treatment of, 2–4
Cancer Adjustment Program, 88
Cancer Call-PAC (People Against
    Cancer), 93
Cancer Care, Inc., 93
Cancer Center of University
    Hospitals At-Home
    Rehabilitation Program, 52
Cancer Information Center, 85
Cancer Information Services (CIS),
    82, 87
Candlelighters Foundation, 95
Candlelighters National
    Headquarters, 56–57
*Candlelighters National Newsletter*, 54
*Candlelighters Teenage Newsletter*, 53
CanSurmount program, 87–88
Caraway, 65
Carbohydrates, 15–16
    foods high in, 61
Cardomom, 65
Cayenne, 65
Center for Attitudinal Healing, 52
Centering Corp., 54
Cheese, 62
Chemotherapy, 5–7
Chemotherapy nurse, 3
"Chemotherapy: Your Weapon
    Against Cancer" (Kulkin,
    Greenspan), 102
Chervil, 66
Chewing, children's difficulty with,
    50
*Childhood Cancer: A Pamphlet for
    Parents* (Sallan and
    Newburger), 54
*Childhood Leukemia: A Pamphlet for
    Parents* (Friedman, Karon, and
    Goldsmith), 58
*Children Die Too* (Johnson and
    Johnson), 54
*Children in Hospitals, Inc.*
    (Newsletter), 54–55, 57
Children with cancer, 44–59
    feeding problems of, 48–51
    information for parents of, 54–59
    information for siblings of, 53–
    54

Children with cancer, *continued*
    nutritional status of, 44–45
    nutrition program for, 45–46
    parents of, 47, 54–59
    programs for, 95–96
    reading material for, 51–59
    snacks for, 51
Chili powder, 66
Chilton, L., 104
Chives, 66
*Choices* (Morra and Pohs), 99
Cinnamon, 66
Clear liquid diet, 235
Clinical nurse specialist, 3
Cloves, 66
Colostomy, 31, 32
Comprehensive Cancer Centers,
    84–86
Constipation, 25, 30
Convenience foods, adding extra
    nutrition to, 62
Cooking, 75–76
Cooking utensils, 23
*Coping at Home with Cancer. For
    Parents by a Parent* (Cottrell), 54
*Coping with Prolonged Health
    Impairment in Your Child*
    (McCollum), 55
Coriander, 66
Corn muffin mix, 63
Cottrell, N., 55
Cramping, 29–30
Cream
    whipped, 60
    *see also* Sour cream
Cumin, 66
Curry, 66

Dental problems, taste alterations
    and, 23
Detoxification, 81
Diarrhea, 19, 29–30, 77
    in children with cancer, 50
    in colostomy and ileostomy
    patients, 32
Diet
    clear liquid, 235
    fiber-restricted, 242–44
    lactose-free, 237
    moderately restricted sodium, 236

"Diet Guide for Chemotherapy Patients, A" (Ellis Fischel State Cancer Hospital), 103
*Diet and Nutrition: A Resource for Parents of Children with Cancer,* 59
"Dietary Tips for Possible Nutrition-Related Problems in the Pediatric Cancer Patient" (Moore), 104
Dietitian (nutritionist), 3
Digestion of food, 17–19
Dill, 66
"Diseases of the Colon and Rectum" (American Medical Association), 101
Dobos, J. A., 52
Drasin, H., 98–99
Dry mouth, 24

Edema (water retention), 33
Eggs, 67
Electrolytes, 6–7
Elimination of waste products, 19
Ellis Fischel State Cancer Hospital, 103
*Emotional Aspects of Childhood Cancer and Leukemia: A Handbook for Parents* (Spinetta, Spinetta, Kung, and Schwartz), 55
"Esophagostomy or Pharyngostomy Tube Feeding" (Olson), 100
Esophagus, 41
Exercise, between meals, 26

Fat-restricted diet, 239
Fats, 15
Fennel, 66
Fiber, dietary:
    content of selected foods, 241–242
    low-fiber diet, 242–244
Fish, 62
Fishman, J., 99
Flumnerfelt, P., 57
"Food for Those Who Hesitate . . . Tips that They Might Tolerate" (Helsel), 103
Food groups, 11

Food preparation, *see* Cooking
Freezing food, 64
Friedman, B., 58
Friends, 73–74
Fullness, feeling of, 25–26

Gas, 32
Gastrointestinal (GI) tract, 17
    cancer of, 39–43
Ginger, 67
Goldsmith, G., 58
Government Printing Office, U.S., 57, 59
*Guide to Good Nutrition During and After Chemotherapy and Radiation, A* (Aker and Lenssen), 99

*Health Through Nutrition: A Comprehensive Guide for the Cancer Patient* (Rosenbaum, Stitt, Drasin, and Rosenbaum), 98–99
Helsel, J. E., 103
Herbs, 64, 65–69
    using, 70
High carbohydrate diet, pancreatic function and, 43
"High Protein Soft Diet" (pamphlet), 100
Holleg, A. I., 99
*Home Care for Dying Children: A Manual for Parents* (Moldow and Martinson), 55
"Home Care Guide for Patients with Head and Neck Disease" (pamphlet), 100
*Hospital Days—Treatment Ways* (Warmbier), 51

I Can Cope program, 87–88
Ileostomy, 31, 32
Immunotherapy, 8–9
Information, 84–105
    from American Cancer Society, 87–91
    from Cancer Information Services, 87
    for children with cancer and their families, 51–59

Information, *continued*
  from Comprehensive Cancer
    Centers, 84–86
  on low-sodium diets, 104
  from national and regional
    education and self-help
    organizations, 91–95
  on nutrition, 98–105
International Association for
  Enterostomal Therapy, 32
International Association of
  Laryngectomies, 92
Intestinal tract, 42
Iron, 42

Johnson, B. L., 98
Johnson, J., 54
Johnson, S. M., 54

Karon, M., 58
Khosness, J. A., 52
Kung, F., 55

Lact-Aid, 34
Lactose-free dairy substitutes, 34
Lactose-free diet, 237
Lactose intolerance, 33–34
Laetrile, 81
Large intestine, 42
Lederer, B., 56
Lenssen, P., 99
*Leukemia: A Guide to the Management
  of the Disease* (Taylor), 58
*Leukemia and the Family* (brochure)
  58
Leukemia Society of America, 55,
  58, 92
Liquid formulas, 36–38
  manufacturers of, 244–246
Little, Brown and Co., 55
*Living One Day At a Time (LODAT).
  Oncology Handbook for Parents*
  (Lederer), 56
"Looking Forward . . . A
  Guidebook for the
  Laryngectomee" (Keith,
  Shane, Coates, Devine), 101
Low-fiber diet, 242–244
Low-sodium diet, 33, 236
  information on, 104

Macaroni and cheese, 6*t*
McCollum, A. T., 55
Mace, 67
Make Today Count, 92
Margarine, 61
Marjoram, 67
Marshall, C. U., 57
Martinson, I. M., 55
Mayonnaise, 61
Meat, 62
  loss of appetite for, 23
Medications
  pain, 35
  taste sensation and, 23
Medium chain triglycerides (MCT),
  43
Megavitamins, 82
Memorial Sloan-Kettering Cancer
  Center, 104
Metallic taste, 22, 23
Milk and milk products:
  dry milk powder, 62
  fortified, 62
  *see also* Lactose intolerance
Minerals, 16
Mineral supplements, 16–17
Mini-meals, 25–26
Mint, 67
Mister Rogers, 58
Moldow, D. G., 55
Morra, M., 98, 99
Mouth:
  cancer of, 39
  dry, 24
  sore, 24–25, 40
Mouth blindness, 22, 39
Mouth sores (stomatitis or
  mucositis), 31, 51
Mouthwashes, 23, 31
Mustard, 67

"Naso-Gastric Tube Feeding"
  (Olson), 101
National Cancer Institute, 79
  Office of Cancer
    Communications, 52, 58, 59,
    84
  publications from, 96–98
National Foundation for Ileitis and
  Colitis, The, 92

National Hospice Organization, 93
National Self-Help Clearing House, 93
Nausea, 21–22, 26–28, 77
  in children with cancer, 49–50
Newberger, P., 54
Nutmeg, 67
Nutrients, 10–17
Nutrition, 4–5
  information sources on, 98–105
"Nutrition: A Helpful Ally in Cancer Therapy" (pamphlet), 99–100
"Nutritional Concerns . . . for Troubled Eaters During Radiation Therapy to the Head and Neck Areas" (Memorial Sloan-Kettering Cancer Center), 104
"Nutritional Guide for Patients Receiving Upper and Lower Abdominal Radiation Therapy" (Persigehl), 103
Nutritional information centers, 94
"Nutrition During and After Radiation Therapy and Chemotherapy" (Williams), 104
"Nutrition for Patients Receiving Chemotherapy and Radiation Treatment" (American Cancer Society), 102–103
Nutritionist (dietitian), 3
Nuts, 61

Occupational therapist, 3
Odor of food, nausea and, 27
Olson, M. L., 100, 101
Oncologist, 3
Onions, 64
"On Nutrition and Liquid Diet" (Olson), 103
Oral cavity, surgery in, 39
Oregano, 67
*Organization and Information Handbook for Parents Groups: 1977–1978*, 56
Ostomies, 31–32
Overeating, 32–33

Pain, 34–35
Pain clinics, 94–95
Pain control referral groups, 94
Pain medication, 35
Pancreas, 42–43
Pancreatic enzymes, 81
Parents, of children with cancer, 47, 54–59
*Parents: When Your Preschooler is Hospitalized, Consider Yourself an Important Member of the Medical Team* (Saphier), 57
Parsley, 68
Peanut butter, 62
*Pediatric Oncology Bibliography* (Sachs and Tharp), 57
Pendleton, Edity, 53
Pharmacist, 3
Physical limitations or disabilities, 38
Physical therapist, 3
Pizzo, P. D., 58
Pohs, E., 99
Poppy seed, 68
Poultry, 62
"Progressive Blenderized Diet" (pamphlet), 102
Protein:
  providing extra, 61–62
  snacks high in, 63–64
Psychiatric social worker, 3
Psychiatrist, 3
Psychologist, 3
Publications, 96–105
  from the National Cancer Insitute, 96–98
  *see also* Information

Radiation therapist, 3
Radiation therapy, 7–8
*Radiation Therapy: A Family Handbook* (Marshall and Flumnerfelt), 57
"Radiation Therapy: How It Can Help You" (Chilton), 104
Radiation therapy technologist, 3
Radiologist, 3
Reach to Recovery program, 92
Relatives, 73–74
Relaxing before eating, 26, 76

Rest after eating, 27, 28
"Restricted Fiber Diet" (pamphlet), 102
Ronald McDonald Houses, 95–96
Rosemary, 68
Rosenbaum, E. H., 98–99
Rosenbaum, I. R., 98–99
Rudolph, L. A., 52–54

Sachs, M., 56
Saffron, 65
Sage, 65
Saliva substitutes, commercially available, 24, 247
Sallan, S. E., 54, 58
Salt:
  water retention and, 33
  see also Low-sodium diet
Saphier, M. K., 56
Satiety, early, 25–26
Savory, 65
Schiff, H. S., 58
Schwartz, D. B., 55
Sesame, 68
Sherman, M., 59
Siblings, of children with cancer, information for, 53–54
Sidney Farber Cancer Institute, 54, 58
Small intestine, 42
Smell, alterations in, 22–23
Snacks:
  for children, 51
  high-calorie and high-protein, 63–64
"Soft and Blended Foods (for Head and Neck Radiation Patients)" (Persigehl), 102
Solving the Eating Problems of Cancer Patients (Johnson, Morra, Suski), 98
Something's Got to Taste Good: The Cancer Patient's Cookbook (Fishman, Anrod), 99
Sore mouth and throat, 24–25
Sour cream, 61
Spices, 61–69
  using, 70
Spinetta, J., 55
Spinetta, P. D., 55

Stare, Frederick, 11
Stitt, C. A., 98–99
Stomach, surgery or other treatment of, 41–42
Story About Cancer, A (Dobos), 52
Story About Leukemia to Color, A (Tharp, Dobos), 52
Stouffer's Escalloped Chicken and Noodle Casserole, 63
Sugar Lo Company, 34
Surgery, 5
  in oral cavity, 39
Suski, N., 98
Swallowing:
  children's difficulty with, 50
  sore mouth and throat and, 24–25

Talking to Children About Death, 57
Tarragon, 68
Taste, alterations in, 22–23
Taylor, G., 58
Team approach to the treatment of cancer, 4
Teens Newsletter, Candlelighters, 53
Teeth:
  brushing, 25
  see also Dental problems
Temperature of food, 23, 25
Tending the Sick Child (Sherman), 59
Tharp, P. S., 52, 56
There Is a Rainbow Behind Every Dark Cloud, 52
Throat:
  cancer of, 39
  sore, 40
Thyme, 68
Tofu, 62
Tongue, cancer of, 39
Too Old to Cry, Too Young to Die (Pendleton), 53
TOUCH (Today Our Understanding of Cancer is Hope), 93
Treatment of cancer, 2–4
  alternative, 78–83
Treatment days, finding time to eat on, 74

Tube feeding, 35–38, 40–41
  blenderized formula for, 248
Turmeric, 68

UCLA Psychological Telephone
    Counseling Service, 93
United Cancer Council (UCC), 92
United Ostomy Association, 32, 55,
    92
Urostomy, 31

Vitamin B12, 42
Vitamins, 16
Vitamin supplement, 16
Vomiting, 28–29, 77
  in children with cancer, 49–50

*Waiting for Johnny Miracle* (Bach),
    53
Warmbier, J., 51
Waste products, elimination of, 19
Water, 17

Watercress, 68
Water retention (edema), 33
Weight gain, 32–33
*What Happened to You Happened to
    Me* (Kjosness, Rudolph), 52
*What You Need to Know . . . 1979*
    (brochure), 59
*When Your Brother or Sister Has
    Cancer* (Rudolph), 53
*When Your Child Goes to the Hospital,*
    58–59
*When Your Child Goes to the Hospital*
    (Pizzo), 59
Williams, S. M., 104

Yogurt, 62
*You and Leukemia: A Day at a Time*
    (Baker), 52
*You Can Fight Cancer and Win*
    (Brody and Holleg), 99
*Young People with Cancer: A
    Handbook for Parents,* 59

# RECIPE INDEX

Almond sauce, 202
Appetizers:
  cheese ball, 108
  cheese spread, 108
  mushroom and cheese, 109
  steak teriyaki, 171
  turkey nibblers, 112
  *see also* Dip; Snacks; Spread
Apple:
  -cheese snack, 114
  -lime cooler, 121
  salad, zippy, 128–129
  souffle, 217
Apple cider, sparkling, 120
Applesauce:
  cake, 224
  deluxe, 214
  toast, 113
Apricot syrup, 230
Asparagus and egg salad, 130
Avocado soup
  chicken, chilled, 128
  cold cream of, 126

Banana:
  blender, 118
  bread, 138
    best banana nut bread, 140
    cranberry bran, 139
  -cranberry toast, 113

Banana, *continued*
  in sherry, 213
  -strawberry yogurt cooler, 118
Barbecue baked fish, 191
Batter bread, bran, 142
Béarnaise sauce, 160
  blender, 206
Beef:
  'n' beer casserole, 170
  chili, 176
  chili con carne, 170
  meatballs, saucy, 175
  meat loaf, spicy jalapeno, 171
  and mushroom sandwich, 136
  patties in wine sauce, 173
  pot roast, lazy day, 173
  shish kebabs, 174
  stroganoff
    hamburger, 174
    speedy, 175
  *see also* Steak
Beverages:
  apple-lime cooler, 121
  blender banana, 118
  breakfast in a glass, 116
  breakfast shake, 116–117
  cranberry cocktail, 120
  floating rainbow, 121
  fruit juice cocktail, tangy, 120
  glow wine, 119

Beverages, *continued*
   iced coffee, elegant, 119
   meal in a glass, 117
   orange eggnog, 117
   sparkling apple cider, 120
   strawberry-banana yogurt cooler,
     118
   tart tropical fizz, 121
   tropic fizz, 118
   winter warmer, 119
Blackberry syrup, 231
Bob's favorite noodle casserole,
   160–161
Bonus potato soup, 124
Bordelaise sauce, 206
Bourbon pound cake, 224–225
Bran batter bread, 142
Brandy:
   cream, whipped, 230
   -orange sauce, 233
Bread:
   banana, 138
     best banana nut bread, 140
     cranberry bran, 139
   bran batter, 142
   cranberry-banana bran, 139
   high-fiber, 139
   pumpkin-nut, 141
   yogurt honey, 140
   zucchini, 141
   *see also* Muffins
Breakfast in a glass, 116
Breakfast shake, 116–117
Broth, 201
Brown sauce, basic, 207
Burgers Béarnaise, 176
Butter, tasty, 179

Cake:
   applesauce, 224
   carrot, 226–227
   gingerbread, 227
   pound
     bourbon, 224–225
     lemon, 226
     rum, 225
California sauce omelet rolls,
   155
Cantaloupe dip, curried, 111
Carrot cake, 226–27

Cereal:
   granola, 109
   hot, 143
Chantilly:
   cream, 230
   melba, 220
Cheese:
   -apple snack, 114
   bake, 148–49
   ball, 108
   in confetti salad, 129
   creamed eggs with, 156
   eggs with, baked, 157
   -fish bake, 191
   fondue
     baked, 149
     Swiss, 149
   'n' ham pie, 161
   and macaroni, 147
   manicotti, 172
   and mushroom appetizers, 109
   noodle casserole, 164
   and onion pie, 147
   pot de creme, 217
   rarebit, 151
   sauce
     creamy, 202
     for fish, tangy, 202–203
     herb-, 203
     instant, 205
     mornay, 205
     special, 205
   spread, 108
   triangles, Greek feta, 112
   -turkey casserole, 186
Cherry:
   sauce, 168
   syrup, 231
Chicken:
   a la king, 185
   -avocado soup, chilled, 128
   breasts, spicy, 180
   casserole, company, 184
   Chinese, cold, 184
   creamed, 185
   curried
     cold, 183
     orange, 180
   divan, instant, 181
   Italiano, broiled, 178

Chicken, *continued*
  lemon, marinated, 178
  lemon sesame, 179
  piccata, 169
  puff, 150–151
  quiche, 151
  -rice casserole, 181
  salad, crunchy, 130
  summer garden, 182
  sweet-and-sour, 178–179
  tetrazzini, 187
  western, 183
  in wine, effortless, 182
Chili, 176
  con carne, 170
Chiliburger, 176–177
Chocolate:
  -coffee sauce, 233
  mousse pie, 222
Clam(s):
  chowder, easy New England, 124
  sauce, white, 197
Coconut balls, 221
Coffee:
  -chocolate sauce, 233
  iced, elegant, 119
Compote, tropical fruit and wine,
    212–213
Confetti salad, 129
Cookies:
  coconut balls, 221
  peanut butter
    jelly thumbprint, 221
    orange, 221
    sandwich, 221
    spritz, 221
Cottage cheese:
  meat loaf, Katherine's, 177
  pancakes, 144
Crab au gratin, 195
Crabmeat soup, 125
Crackers, oyster, zesty, 115
Cranberry:
  -banana bran bread, 139
  -banana toast, 113
  cocktail, 120
  delight, 122
  salad, 130–131
Cream:
  chantilly, 230
  chantilly melba, 220

Cream, *continued*
  sauce, 200, 201, 205
  whipped brandy, 230
Creole sauce, 204
Creole sauce omelet rolls, 152
Crepes, 222
  suzette, 221
Crisscross potatoes, 164
Cucumber soup, cold, 127
Cumberland sauce, 203
Curry (curried):
  cantaloupe dip, 111
  chicken
    cold, 183
    orange, 180
  dip, 110
  eggs, cold, 158
  sauce, 202

Desserts, 211–228
  applesauce deluxe, 214
  apple souffle, 217
  banana in sherry, 213
  cake
    applesauce, 224
    bourbon pound, 224–225
    carrot, 226
    lemon pound, 226
    rum, 225
  chantilly melba, 220
  cheese pot de creme, 217
  crepes, 222
    suzette, 221
  grapefruit, broiled, 215
  iced fruit, 212
  lemonade fluff, frosty, 218
  macedoine of fruit, 212
  nut bars, 220
  minted pineapple, 214
  peach melba, 216
  peanut butter cookies, 220–221
  peanut butter ice cream balls,
    217
  pie
    chocolate mousse, 222
    pastry for, 228
    pecan, 223
    strawberry-yogurt refrigerator,
      223
  pineapple cream, 218
  raspberry melon boats, 213

Desserts, *continued*
  raspberry-pineapple ice, 216
  rice pudding
    creamy, 219
    old-fashioned, 219
  sherbet
    fruit, 214
    lemon, rich, 216
    strawberry, 215
  spring delight, 215
  tropical fruit and wine compote,
    212–213
Dessert sauces, 229–234
  brandy orange sauce, 233
  chantilly cream, 230
  coffee chocolate sauce, 233
  fruit sundae sauce, 233
  fruit syrups, 230–231
  hard sauce, 231
  melba, blender sauce, 232
    punchy rum sauce, 232
  rum sauce, 231
  sherry or port wine sauce, 232
  whipped brandy cream, 230
Dill-lemon sauce, shrimp with, 197
Dip:
  curried cantaloupe, 111
  curry, 110
  Mexican, 111
  Tex-Mex, 110
  zippy, 111

Easy New England clam chowder,
    124
Egg(s):
  a la king, 156
  and asparagus salad, 130
  baked, 155
    with cheese, 157
    Provencal, 159
  béarnaise, 160
  Benedict, quick, 146
  cheesy creamed, 156
  curried, cold, 158
  foo young, 158
  and fries, 146
  and ham en croute, 162
  salad sandwich, 132
  scrambled, 146
  shirred, with mushrooms, 159
  *see also* Omelet; Souffle

Eggnog, orange, 117
Ever-ready muffins, 138

Feta cheese triangles, Greek, 112
Fettucini carbonara, 161
Fiesta salad, 128
Fish:
  baked, 190
    barbecue, 191
    cheese-, 191
    crusty, 190
  fillets
    saucy, 193
    sweet and sour, 192
  steamed in foil, 194
  tangy cheese sauce for, 202–203
Floating rainbow, 121
Flounder, baked, deluxe, 193
Fondue
  baked cheese, 149
  Swiss, 149
French toast, 142
  with maple-pecan syrup, 143
  orange, 143
Fruit
  iced, 212
  juice cocktail, tangy, 120
  kebab garnish, 173
  macedoine of, 212
  sherbet, 214
  sundae sauce, 233
  syrups, 230–231
  'n' tuna sandwich, 135
  and wine compote, tropical, 212
    213
  *see also specific fruits*

Garnish, kebab, fruit, 173
Giblet gravy, creamy, 207
Gingerbread, 227
Granola, 109
  bars, 114
Grapefruit, broiled, 215
Gravy:
  from canned condensed soup,
    200
  giblet, creamy, 207
  in a hurry, 208
  onion, quick, 207
Greek feta cheese triangles, 112
Glow wine, 119

Haddock, oven-poached, 192
Ham.
  'n' cheese pie, 161
  in confetti salad, 129
  and egg en croute, 162
  in Hawaiian toast sandwich, 131
  and macaroni bake, easy, 163
Hamburger:
  béarnaise, 176
  stroganoff, 174
Hard sauce, 231
Hash, Polynesian, 177
Hawaiian toast sandwich, 131
Herbs:
  butter with, 179
  omelet aux fines herbes, 153
  omelet roll, 154
  sauce, 202
    cheese-, 203
High-fiber bread, 139
Hollandaise sauce, blender, 206
Honey-yogurt bread, 140

Ice:
  raspberry-pineapple, 216
  see also Sherbet
Ice cream:
  balls, peanut butter, 217
  coffee chocolate sauce for, 233
  lemonade fluff, frosty, 218
  sundae sauce for, 233
  see also Sherbet

Jalapeno meat loaf, spicy, 171
Jelly snack, 112–113
Jelly thumbprint cookies, 221

Katherine's cottage cheese meat
    loaf, 177

Lamb shish kebabs, 174
Lazy day pot roast, 173
Lemon:
  chicken
    marinated, 178
    sesame, 179
  -dill sauce, shrimp with, 197
  pound cake, 226
  sherbet, rich, 216
Lemonade fluff, frosty, 218
Lime-apple cooler, 121

Macaroni:
  and cheese, 147
    in Fiesta salad, 128
  and ham bake, easy, 163
  oven, 148
  -tuna-mushroom salad, 129
Macedoine of fruit, 212
Manicotti, 172
Maple-pecan syrup, french toast
    with, 143
Meal in a glass, 117
Meal on a muffin, 131
Meatballs, saucy, 175
Meat loaf:
  cottage cheese, Katherine's, 117
  spicy jalapeno, 171
Meat stock, 201
Melon-raspberry boats, 213
Mexican dip, 111
Minted pineapple, 214
Mousse, chocolate, pie, 222
Mornay sauce, 205
Muffins, ever-ready, 138
Mushroom:
  and beef sandwich, 136
  and cheese appetizers, 109
  omelet, 152–153
  shirred eggs with, 159
  -shrimp sauce, with omelet rolls,
    154–155
  -tuna-macaroni salad, 129
Mustard sauce, 205

Noodle:
  casserole, Bob's favorite, 160–161
  cheese casserole, 164
Nut(s):
  -banana bread, best, 140
  bars, 220
  -pumpkin bread, 141
  sauce, 202

Oats, in granola, 109
Omelet:
  aux fines herbes, 153
  mushroom 152–153
  roll, 154
    California sauce, 155
    Creole sauce, 152
    mushroom-shrimp sauce with,
    154–155

Onion:
   and cheese pie, 147
   gravy, quick, 207
Orange:
   -brandy sauce, 233
   chicken, curried, 180
   in confetti salad, 129
   eggnog, 117
   French toast, 143
   -peanut butter cookies, 221
   squares, 115

Pancakes, cottage cheese, 144
Parsley:
   sauce, 202
   -wine sauce, 204
Pasta, see Fettucini; Macaroni;
     Manicotti; Noodles; Spaghetti
Pea soup, creamy, 126
Peanut butter:
   cookies, 220–221
   ice cream balls, 217
Peach:
   melba, 216
   syrup, 231
Pecans:
   -maple syrup, French toast with,
     143
   pie, 223
   spicy roasted, 108–109
Pepperoni pizza, 135
Piccata, veal or chicken, 169
Pie:
   cheese and onion, 147
   chocolate mousse, 222
   ham 'n' cheese, 161
   pastry for, 228
   pecan, 223
   strawberry-yogurt refrigerator,
     223
   tuna, 194
Pineapple:
   in confetti salad, 129
   in Hawaiian toast sandwich, 131
   minted, 214
   -raspberry ice, 216
   syrup, 230
Pizza:
   quick
     with meat, 133
     no meat, 134

Pizza, continued
   pepperoni, 135
   pick-ups, 134
Polynesian hash, 177
Pork:
   Polynesian hash, 177
   sweet-and-sour, 178–179
Port wine sauce, 232
Potato:
   crisscross, 164
   egg and fries, 146
   soup
     bonus, 124
     chilled, 126
     vichyssoise, 127
Pot de creme, cheese, 217
Pot roast, lazy day, 173
Pound cake:
   lemon, 226
   bourbon, 224–225
Pudding, rice:
   creamy, 219
   old-fashioned, 219
Pumpkin-nut bread, 141
Punchy rum sauce, 232

Quiche:
   chicken, 151
   Lorraine, 152

Raspberry (raspberries):
   -melon boats, 213
   in peach melba, 216
   -pineapple ice, 216
   syrup, 231
Rice:
   -chicken casserole, 181
   pudding
     creamy, 219
     old-fashioned, 219
Roll, omelet, 154
   California sauce, 155
   creole sauce, 152
   mushroom-shrimp sauce with,
     154–155
Rum:
   sauce, 231
     punchy, 232
   cake, 225

Salad:
    apple, zippy, 128–129
    chicken, crunchy, 130
    confetti, 129
    cranberry, 130–131
    egg, sandwich, 132
    egg and asparagus, 130
    fiesta, 128
    tuna-mushroom-macaroni, 129
Salmon sandwich, open-faced, 135
Sandwich(es):
    beef and mushroom, 136
    egg salad, 132
    fruit 'n' tuna, 135
    Hawaiian toast, 131
    Meal on a muffin, 131
    salmon, open-faced, 135
    seafood, hot, 132
    Sloppy Joe, 133
Sauce:
    almond, 202
    béarnaise, 160
        blender, 206
    bordelaise, 206
    brown, basic, 207
    California, omelet rolls with, 155
    canned condensed soups used
        for, 200–201
    cheese
        creamy, 202
        for fish, tangy, 202–203
        instant, 205
        mornay, 205
        special, 205
    cherry, 168
    cream, 205
    creole, 204
        omelet rolls, 152
    Cumberland, 203
    dessert, see Dessert sauces
    herb, 202
    herb-cheese, 203
    hollandaise, blender, 206
    lemon-dill, shrimp with, 197
    mornay, 205
    mushroom-shrimp, with omelet
        rolls, 154–155
    mustard, 205
    nut, 202
    parsley, 202

Sauce, *continued*
    Swedish, 204
    tomato, 200
    white, 208
    white clam, 197
    wine, beef patties in, 173
    see also Gravy
Scrambled eggs, 146
Seafood:
    newburg, 195
    sandwiches, hot, 132
Sesame seeds, lemon chicken with,
    179
Sherbet:
    fruit, 214
    lemon, rich, 216
    strawberry, 215
Sherry:
    banana in, 213
    sauce, 232
Shish kebabs, 174
Shrimp:
    with lemon-dill sauce, 197
    -mushroom sauce with omelet
        rolls, 154–155
    supreme, 198
Sloppy joe, 133
Snacks:
    apple-cheese, 114
    applesauce toast, 113
    cranberry banana toast, 113
    crisp toast, 116
    granola, 109
    granola bars, 114
    jelly, 112–113
    nut bars, 220
    packs, 114–115
    pecans, spicy roasted, 108
    see also Sandwich(es)
Souffle:
    apple, 217
    baked, 148
    basic, 150
    oven, 157
Soup:
    avocado, cold cream of, 126
    chicken-avocado, chilled, 128
    chilled, easy (condensed), 127
    condensed canned, uses for, 200–
        201

Soup, *continued*
  crabmeat, 125
  cream of spinach, 125
  cucumber, cold, 127
  New England clam chowder,
    easy, 124
  pea, creamy, 126
  potato
    bonus, 124
    chilled, 126
    vichyssoise, 127
  toppers for, 124
  vegetable, hearty, 125
Spaghetti, chicken or turkey
  tetrazzini with, 187
Spinach:
  best-ever, 162
  soup, cream of, 125
  supreme, 165
Spread, cheese, 108
Spring delight, 215
Steak:
  au poivre, 172
  teriyaki, 171
Stock, 201
Strawberry (strawberries):
  -banana yogurt cooler, 118
  sherbet, 215
  spring delight, 215
  syrup, 230
  -yogurt refrigerator pie, 223
Swedish sauce, 204
Sweet-and-sour chicken or pork,
  178
Sweet and sour fish fillets, 192
Swiss fondue, 149

Tarragon veal, 168
Tex-Mex dip, 110
Toast:
  applesauce, 113
  crisp, 116
  cranberry banana, 113
  french, *see* French toast
Toasty turkeywiches, 132–133
Tomato sauce, 200

Topping for vegetables, 209
Tropical fizz, tart, 121
Tropical fruit and wine compote,
  212–213
Tropic fizz, 118
Tuna:
  casserole, 196
  'n' fruit sandwich, 135
  a la king, 196
  -mushroom-macaroni salad, 129
  pie, 194
Turkey:
  -cheese casserole, 186
  nibblers, 112
  stroganoff, 186
  tetrazzini, 187
Turkeywiches, toasty, 132–133

Veal:
  cutlet Parmesan, 169
  piccata, 169
  tarragon, 168
Vegetable(s):
  soup, hearty, 125
  topping, 209
Vichyssoise, 127

Western chicken, 183
White clam sauce, 197
White sauce, 200, 201, 208
Wine:
  compote, tropical fruit and, 212–
    213
  glow, 119
  -parsley sauce, 204
  sauce, beef patties in, 173
Winter warmer, 119

Yogurt:
  cooler, strawberry banana, 118
  -honey bread, 140
  -strawberry refrigerator pie,
    223

Zippy dip, 109
Zucchini bread, 141